NO-NONSENSE GUIDE TO

CHOLESTEROL MEDICATIONS

INFORMED CONSENT AND STATIN DRUGS

A SmartMEDinfo Book by

Moira Dolan, M.D.

OTHER BOOKS

*No-Nonsense Guide to Psychiatric Drugs, Including
Mental Effects of Common Non-Psych Medications*

No-Nonsense Guide to Antibiotics, Dangers, Benefits & Proper Use

Dedicated to Duane Edgar Graveline, MD, MPH, physician, NASA astronaut, United States Air Force (USAF) research scientist, and the very first to alert the public about the adverse effects of statin drugs. See more at www.spacedoc.com.

TABLE OF CONTENTS

CHAPTER 1

WHY GET INFORMED?

In order to make a rational decision about taking statin drugs or not, a person needs to be aware of pertinent information:

What is a statin?

How do statins work?

What is known and not known about how well statin drugs work?

What is known and not known about statin safety and hazards?

What are the alternatives to taking statins?

What conflicts of interest are inherent in the recommendation for you to take statins?

A 2015 study sheds some light on these blockbuster-selling drugs:[1]

- For people with no previous cardiovascular event, survival data covered a range from dying 5 days earlier than those not on statins to living 19 days longer than people not on a statin. The numbers averaged out to a whopping 3.2 days longer survival for statin users. Keep in mind that these patients were on statins daily for years in order to average this half a week survival advantage.

- For people who'd already had a cardiovascular event, the comparative survival range for statin users was death 10 days earlier compared to non-users of statins to living 27 days longer compared to those not on a statin. This averaged to a survival advantage of 4.1 days resulting from the years and years they were on the statin drug.

3 to 4 additional days of life in exchange for years of statin treatment and drug side effects!

This information has been lying around in the study data all along. It came out of a comprehensive review of all 26 of the major studies on statin drugs. It turns out that only 11 of them adequately reported on survival statistics. These 11 studies totaled over 85,000 patients, and covered 5 bestselling statin drugs.

It is interesting that it is coming to light only when all major statin drugs have expired patents. And just by coincidence, brand new cholesterol lowering drugs have just been FDA approved. PCSK9 inhibitors cost up to $14,000 per year and are newly patented with no risk of generic competition for 20 years. These drugs, Praluent and Repatha, have so far not been claimed to save lives, only to dramatically lower cholesterol.

A person should only consent to taking a statin drug after gaining a full understanding of the facts and implications of their decision. Without this due diligence, the individual could really be in for some serious, yet preventable, drug side effects. In other words, will statins be beneficial to you and worth the side effect risks?

Ever hear about some relative who went loopy, suffered a fall, then died while under a doctor's care and taking 13 prescribed medications?

No Informed Consent!

The *No-Nonsense* series gives drug information often not shared by your doctor and not easy to extract from sites like webmd, Dr. Google, or Wikipedia. Statin drugs are likely the most over-prescribed, least effective powders ever marketed, and this guide provides informed consent information you should consider before taking them.

Per the official legal definition, Informed Consent requires the patient be in possession of their faculties, meaning not mentally incompetent.

In today's health care system, it is almost never mental incompetence inhibiting rational medical decision-making. [2] Some patients may feel social pressures, ridicule, or financial pressures; or fear being labelled "non-compliant" for not following doctor's orders or questioning popular medical trends. The usual seven-minute patient-doctor face-to-face visit can also prevent the opportunity for real informed consent.

But most of the time, lack of informed consent is because of a combination of ignorance and low ethics. Sadly, most patients do not know about their legal right to informed consent, and most physicians feel no ethical responsibility to provide it. Doctors in a busy practice don't go home and read medical journals about the actual facts, figures, and side effects of drugs, and rarely ever with a critical eye, if they do. Most do not challenge the latest drug news supplied by pharmaceutical marketing divisions, but rather depend on the steady stream of drug company promotional material to tell them what treatments they should offer.

The Western tradition of medical ethics dates back to Hippocrates, a Greek physician from about 500 BC. His writings are the earliest Greek medical documents known and include the famous Hippocratic Oath. There are many translations of what is believed to be the original oath scribed by Hippocrates. Classical versions are an oath to the gods and include promises to honor one's teacher, pass on one's medical knowledge, apply nutritional remedies, refrain from using or suggesting deadly drugs, refuse to participate in abortion, leave surgery to the surgeons, maintain patient confidentiality, and never engage in sexual relations with a patient. It is generally interpreted as simply keeping the patient's best interests at heart. [3]

It may come as a shock that medical schools do *not* have any requirement for graduating doctors to take the oath. When the Oath is read at an *optional* convocation ceremony, most have taken the liberty of modifing the original Oath. Popular revisions include dropping the opening vow to the gods, omitting any reference to prohibition against abortion, and qualifying the ban on sexual activity with patients. In short, this ethical guide has been dropped or watered down to fit modern morals, or amorality, as the case may be.

The Oath has been popularly summarized as meaning "first do no harm," which is a phrase that does not actually appear in the classical version. The promise to refrain from using deadly drugs is the true predecessor to informed consent.

Knowing all drugs have some potential for adverse effects, how does the modern day physician adhere to the oath to refrain from giving or suggesting deadly drugs? The practice of providing informed consent is the closest medcial practitioners come to really applying the ethical code the oath is meant to represent. Unfortunately, most physicians don't genuinely give the opportunity for informed consent despite national guidelines, state level legislation, and medical board policies that require informed consent to varying degrees.

Medical ethics codes through the 19th century strictly dealt with the physician's opinion of what *he* thought was best for the patient. Obtaining the patient's consent was not addressed directly until the aftermath of WWII. The Nuremberg Trials involved testimony on the atrocities committed by members of the Nazi Party in the name of medical science. Criminal proceedings were held for 23 physicians and administrators who carried out the Nazi regime's political objectives on the pretext of medical treatments, including eugenics, euthanasia, and experimentation. The court's proceedings heard 85 witnesses and evaluated some 1500 documents. While the findings of criminality focused on the deeds committed as 'acts of duty' during wartime, the investigations encompassed civilian and pre-war conduct as well.

These guys were bad news. What they got away with was so creepy that the rest of the world decided they needed to agree on some basic medical ethics guidelines in order to protect patients. The *Nuremberg Directives for Human Experimentation* was composed, usually referred to as the *Nuremberg Code.* The Code specifies that participants can consent to human experimentation only after full information is divulged and they have been given an opportunity to evaluate it. It also states that consent should be entirely voluntary and free of coercion. The information should be given to the patient in a comprehensible way with the intention of truly enlightening the potential participant, and should include data on "all inconveniences, hazards...and effects on his health or person" that may result from the treatment. [4]

A refinement of the *Nuremberg Code* occurred with the *Declaration of Helsinki*, an ethics policy of the World Medical Association. It was first adopted in 1964 in Helsinki, Finland and revised many times since. The *Declaration* modernizes the concepts dealt with in the *Nuremberg Code* and expands on the basic principles. It addresses ethical standards that promote respect for all human beings and protects their health and human rights during medical experimentation. It calls for subjects to be informed before voluntarily submitting to any treatment. [5]

The *Helsinki Declaration* also extends the concept of experimentation to include the usual practice of clinical medicine. It implies there can be unintended, disregarded, covert, or overt human experimentation well outside the bounds of a research program; for example, *off-label* applications (giving a drug to someone for other than what their country's drug regulating agenices approved it for). The Food and Drug Administarition (FDA) is the United States' national drug regulating body. It is a direct violation of the *Helsinki Declaration* when drugs for off-label applications are prescribed in the absence of informed consent; i.e., patients are not told by their doctors that the FDA has not approved the drug for their specific condition.

The *Belmont Report* is a uniquely American ethical code for informed consent, which it calls for in everyday practice, as well as traditional research environments. It also expressly includes mental treatments. Belmont emphasizes that the patient is to be given adequate information on risks and benefits, and in a way so as to be comprehended by the recipient. Any consent to treatment must be entirely voluntary. The implication in the *Belmont Report* is that a person is not really voluntarily consenting to treatment when he or she has not been given adequate information with which to make such a decision. A person should have the concept of informed consent in mind during every single medical interaction. [6]

Doctors are supposed to obtain agreement to any course of treatment, and in order to do so, they must tell their patient anything that may substantially affect their decision. In a world where they don't serve peanuts on the plane if one passenger mentions a peanut allergy, one would think it would be routine for doctors to inform patients when the drug they are recommending can cause dementia or cancer!

The information provided here is an interpretation of information on statin drugs that is also widely available to physicians. This is not intended to be a comprehensive nor exhaustive review of everything known in any quarter about statin drugs. It is provided as supplement to patient/doctor discussions in order to facilitate informed consent.

CHAPTER 2

What is Cholesterol?

Cholesterol is a type of fat with many important roles. The most basic of these is acting as one of the building blocks of cells.

The word comes from the Greek *khole–* meaning "bile." Bile is nothing more than cholesterol juice that aids proper digestion. It is the greenish yellow fluid made by your liver. Bile is stored in the gall bladder, a small sack tucked under the liver. The next part of the word is from the Greek *–stereos* meaning "stiff." Cholesterol consists of four fused rings of carbon with a single oxygen molecule sticking out the end. Biochemists call anything with a similar structure a *sterol.* Just like beef fat floating in a soup bowl, sterols cannot be dissolved in water.

Cholesterol is made in the liver and concentrated in the gall bladder. The cholesterol in bile helps break down fats and oil you eat into smaller particles so the body can absorb them. Bile is needed to absorb vitamins from food that cannot be dissolved in water, such as vitamins A, D, E, and K. Bile is also dumped into the gut as a way to rid the body of too much cholesterol.

Life as we know it could not exist if not for sterols. All animals have sterols, many of them identical to our human cholesterol. Even insects and plants have sterols. Cholesterol is needed for cells to function normally and to keep cell membranes stable and flexible. It is the starting molecule for many hormones, including the sex hormones estrogen, testosterone, and progesterone, and is used to make the stress-response hormone *cortisol,* which also plays a role in regulating blood sugar and the body's response to infection. Cholesterol is the foundation for the lesser-known hormone *aldosterone,* which regulates salt and water in the bloodstream. It attaches to the inactive form of pre-vitamin D to make it into activated vitamin D, essential to bone strength, tooth growth, and prevention of heart disease and cancer.

Your body knows how much cholesterol it needs to keep all these important roles filled and monitors amounts with the liver. The liver has an automatic feedback loop, such that it will decrease its own production of cholesterol when more cholesterol-rich foods are eaten. It will ramp cholesterol production back up when eating a low-fat diet.

It is estimated that some 25% of the body's cholesterol is in the brain. Aside from being a structural component of brain cells, it facilitates everything from speed of nerve impulses to brain cell growth and repair.

Despite everything known about cholesterol and how it works, there is a lot even the most knowledgeable research scientists cannot answer. The body is a beautiful, complex machine we are just now starting to unravel. The cutting edge of modern medications is usually just a sledgehammer approach to repairing a delicately balanced Swiss clock. The approach may knock something back in place, but often with unintended consequences days, months, or years down the road.

Cholesterol levels and the effects of medications that alter those levels means different things for different people. With all of the important roles cholesterol plays, I hope you are starting to get the idea that you should question your doctor's blanket recommendation that "everyone needs to take cholesterol-lowering medications."

How can you be comfortable in knowing you've made an informed decision?

Read on!

CHAPTER 3

HEART HEALTH IN AMERICA

Here's some good news: Americans are living longer. Life expectancy in the United States in 2011 was up to an all-time high of 78.7 years—76 years for men, 81 years for women. This is welcome news, but did you know it still only gives America a ranking of 26th in the world? That's pretty far down the list despite the fact that we spent the most on healthcare of any country in the world. Let's take a deeper look at how this could be.

Deaths from heart disease in the US are higher than twenty-one other countries.

Deaths from cancer are worse than nine other countries.

We are in the worst one-third for deaths from car accidents, the health of our infants, and for how many Americans get dementia.

We have a higher suicide rate than about half the nations of the world.

So what's the deal here? Analysis by the Organization for Economic Cooperation and Development (OECD) lists many factors contributing to the relatively poor US ranking. Among other things, they cite excessive use of prescription drugs as a main factor.

Fact: in the US, we spend two and a half times more per person on health care, and far outstrip the others in how much we spend on prescription drugs per person than the average for all the other countries surveyed! [1]

So we spend more money, take more medication, and yet we die sooner. But here's the kicker: when surveyed about our own perception of how healthy we are, Americans ranked their health care number one.

What is going on here? Are we being led to believe all of this money we spend on health care and wonder drugs is really working? Because the stats show that is not true at all! In fact, countries that *decreased* their per-person spending on pharmaceuticals in the last 4 years are the same ones who have shown a much better rise in life expectancy than the US. [2]

Yes, you read that right!

more prescriptions = shorter lifespan; fewer prescriptions = longer life

The three most likely causes of death in US elderly are heart disease, cancer, and stroke. Two of these, heart disease and stroke, are often lumped together in the term "cardiovascular" to include the heart and all things related to blood vessels. Despite its ranking, the death rate from cardiovascular disease has actually gone down 43% over the last 20 years.

What is causing the improvement in cardiovascular health?

Was the decrease in the US cardiovascular death rate due to the use of cholesterol-lowering medications?

The drug makers would like you to think so, but it does not work that way. Here are the actual statistics:

1994: About 12% of adults were on cholesterol-lowering drugs in 1994;

2004: Use of cholesterol-lowering drugs increased to about 41% of adults;

Comparison 1994 to 2004: In spite of 4 out of every 10 adults taking a cholesterol lowering drug, it turns out the ratio of people with high levels of 'bad' cholesterol *stayed just about the same* from 1994 through 2004.

2011: Use of cholesterol lowering drugs dropped: only 25% age 45 and over were on them in a time period when the heart disease death rate continued to decrease. The 2011 population statistics show that in general, Americans are achieving lower cholesterol numbers, but when a smaller percent are taking cholesterol-lowering medications!

There are so many factors affecting cardiovascular death rate and overall longevity that it is unlikely any one thing would be found responsible for the improvements. For example, the deaths from heart disease went down during a time when *trans* fats were largely removed from fast foods; meanwhile, the consumption of organic foods increased steadily, and people were more likely to quit smoking than to start smoking.

A closer scrutiny of the relationship of cholesterol levels with longevity gives a very different picture than what you may see advertized on TV or promoted by your doctor. A landmark study established that elderly people with higher cholesterol levels tend to live longer. This study looked at the cholesterol levels in 734 elderly with a median age of 89 years—not surprisingly, 642 of them died over the course of the 10-year follow up. Death rates were compared to cholesterol levels. There was a direct relationship of living longer if cholesterol was higher. This and other studies of cholesterol in the elderly show that lowering cholesterol cannot be claimed as a way to prolong life.

What did these old folks die from? The major cause of deaths was heart disease, but the chance of dying from a heart problem was the same no matter the cholesterol levels. In other words, cholesterol level did not in any way predict death from heart disease in this age group. On the flip side, the people with intermediate or low cholesterol levels were more likely to die from infection and cancer. [4]

These facts turn the whole "bad cholesterol" theory on its head.

Are we giving cholesterol-lowering drugs to elderly people who don't need them and completely missing the younger ones who may benefit? Or is it that the drugs don't work as well as big-pharma would like us to believe? Could it be the drugs are causing something else to happen and lowering cholesterol is just an incidental side effect? Is there something else driving down the cardiovascular death rate?

CHAPTER 4

CHOLESTEROL AND THE HEART

The average age for a first heart attack in US men is 65. For women, the age frames are shifted to about five years older with an average age of first heart attack at 70. [1]

The first method ever used to study heart disease was conducting autopsies on people who died of heart attack. Semi-hard plaques were found in many of the subjects, and the plaques were found to consist of cholesterol, calcium, and clotted blood. It was also noticed that rarely, some families of heart attack victims included many relatives who inherited a severe form of very high cholesterol. Those who were stuck with the bad genes dropped dead of heart attacks when they were still quite young. With these two observations, it was logical to conclude that high cholesterol caused blockage of arteries and, in turn, caused death from heart attacks. Without much further research, pharmaceutical companies got to work on drugs that would lower cholesterol. If they could sell this to the public, it would be a huge profit generator.

As laboratory analysis became more sophisticated it was discovered there were many different types of cholesterol. These are categorized according to how dense they are. *High density cholesterol* is the form of cholesterol being carried *out* of the blood stream and into the liver for disposal or recycling. Despite the name, "high density" particles do not contribute to artery blockage. It turns out that high-density cholesterol particles are not part of the problem, but in fact seem to *protect* against heart attacks.

The *low-density,* or less tightly packed cholesterol, has the job of taking cholesterol *into* the cells. Low-density cholesterol can build up in hard plaques on the inner walls of arteries, and it seems to be the kind of cholesterol related to heart attacks. However, it is not a black and white situation because many with elevated low-density type cholesterol never suffer heart disease. I hope you are starting to get the picture that cholesterol, high density or low density, does not play the leading role in the drama of heart disease.

Further sophistication in measuring techniques led to the discovery that low-density cholesterol comes in different sizes, and only the very smallest of low density particles may be the culprits in hardening of the arteries.

Finally, it was found that cholesterol is carried around the body as a complex structure of part fat (also called *lipids*) and part protein. The combination of the words created a new term, *lipoprotein.* High-density lipoprotein, HDL, is good for you; low-density lipoprotein, LDL, can be problematic if it's in the bloodstream at high levels. Another LDL-like particle is lipoprotein (a), abbreviated Lp(a). When this little player was studied in the test tube, it was discovered that its main job is to repair cells and cellular elements, yet it is the single component of cholesterol that has the most to do with forming plaques on artery walls and promoting clots. It seems like Lp(a)'s repair activities can get out of hand and do more harm than good.

Cholesterol is an amazing substance essential to the life of every cell in the body, so it remains a mystery how it could be suddenly discovered to be so bad. Cholesterol evolved with the human body, and the only big changes were external: *in our diets.* Heart disease is an affliction of modern industrialized nations. Cholesterol plaques did not seem to be a major health factor in prehistory or in the pre-industrialized period.

Today we enjoy an abundance of refined carbohydrates—breads, pastas, cereals, rice, and corn. Digestion breaks carbohydrates down into basic sugars the body can use. Some carbohydrates, like table sugar, are simple and go directly into the bloodstream as sugar. Some are more complex and take longer to break down into sugar. Complex carbohydrates, like whole grains and leafy greens, are relatively good for the body because they don't "spike" blood sugar like simple carbs do.

The phenomenon of large-scale food processing combined with the need to promote sales led to the discovery that people will consume more if there is more sugar in packaged foods, and in fact will come to crave sweeteners and carbohydrates. In this way, simple carbs and sugars have entered our everyday diet in much greater quantity than is good for our bodies. Read the label on packaged foods to prove this to yourself.

Sweeteners are a prominent ingredient in ketchup, bread, and peanut butter even though we don't consider those sweet foods.

Now start reading labels on everything you put into your body, but be mindful that when sugar itself is not plainly on the label, you may find some of the other 257 names for sugars, often in unrecognizable chemical terms.

Yet the 'bad fat' theory was pushed so hard by those with a profitable drug to sell that it encouraged health authorities to take up an aggressive anti-fat campaign, and soon all fats got swept into the 'bad' category. We were told to avoid eggs, butter, bacon, and all things deliciously fat. This campaign ignored the abundant evidence pointing to carbs as a far more significant health hazard than fats.

Fat is the ingredient in foods most responsible for giving the feeling that a person has eaten enough; fat gives not just fullness, but more of a sense of satisfaction. Without fat, the body craves carbohydrates and pure sugar. That is exactly why people gain weight when they are on low-fat/high-carb diets. Unfortunately, an excess of simple carbohydrates sets up inflammation in the body. An excess of carbohydrates provokes cells to pour out proteins that irritate the body. When simple carbs are eaten as a greater proportion of each meal, the body is more or less constantly inflamed. A state of inflammation consists of a cascade of biochemical events designed to protect and repair, but can easily go overboard. Effects can range from swelling and excess blood flow to the release of biochemicals that irritate and damage body structures.

In the blood vessels, this type of inflammation activates Lp(a), normally with well-intentioned repair activities. When there is chronic inflammation, Lp(a) activity is thought to get out of hand, then finally tip over into destruction in the walls of blood vessels [2] Imagine a friendly cop going to break up a fight during a parade (the healthy response of the body to unwanted or damaging factors) and then quickly escalating into a full scale riot squad spraying firehoses and rocksalt into the peaceable crowd (inflammation gone overboard).

Remember, the liver will make more cholesterol when the diet does not supply it. The low-fat/high-carb way of eating actually causes blood LDL levels to *rise*. Excess carbs appear to set up an inflammatory condition in the blood vessel walls, and this provokes Lp(a) to go fight a vague enemy called "general inflammation." It is easy to imagine innocent bystanders (the blood vessels) getting mixed up in this war.

At this time, step back and look at the initial theory again:

It was assumed high cholesterol caused blocked arteries. Today's evidence suggests it is actually the other way around.

1. The inflamed artery causes the body's repair systems to go into action against a vague but pervasive threat.

2. The inflammatory actions of carbs in particular seem to push Lp(a) into action.

3. It appears Lp(a) senses the inflammation caused by excessive carbs and springs into action on blood vessels.

4. When this process happens over and over, it is possible that it is overdone and soon a plaque begins to build up.

5. The theory is that eventually the artery is narrowed and clots off entirely.

6. This of course causes a heart attack or a stroke.

Let's use an analogy to illustrate this. Imagine a neighborhood street being the blood vessel. A street party is in progress. It is becoming a little rowdy with too many carbs. A call is made for reinforcements and the liver responds by making and sending more LDL to the area. The party is now getting out of hand (more inflammation), so neighbors call the cops: Lp(a) to the rescue! The Lp(a) cops show up in riot gear and use excessive force, arresting everyone. Even though the Lp(a) thinks it is there to repair something, it is actually further irritating the vessel wall. Some of the party carbs are injured by the Lp(a) cops, and EMS is called. The blood vessel street clogs with ambulances, and there is your clotted off artery.

Saying cholesterol causes plaque and clotting in arteries is like saying crooked joints lead to arthritis. In that case, all we would need to do is straighten out the joints and the arthritis would go away. Of course, we know crooked joints are the *consequence* of arthritis and not the cause. In another example, if someone has gall stone attacks, then calcium can deposit in a thin shell lining the inside of the gall bladder. It would not be advisable to remove all calcium from that person! We know calcium is not the cause of the attacks, but is instead the consequence of repeated inflammation.

It has been convenient to go after one small risk factor—cholesterol—and to generalize it as being a major risk to all people. This line of thinking certainly sells drugs. In the coming chapters we will explore who exactly benefits, and at what cost to those who don't.

CHAPTER 5

WHAT IS A STATIN?

As early as the 1950s, researchers began scrambling to discover ways to treat cholesterol based on the 'bad fat' theory. It was noticed that people who had plenty of vitamin B3 (niacin) in the foods they ate tended to have lower cholesterol levels. Niacin was safely given in high doses to people with a family history of premature heart disease, and it definitely helped lower cholesterol. However, two things about niacin made it unattractive to pharmaceutical companies. At the start of treatment and every time the dose was increased, niacin caused an uncomfortable but totally harmless flushing of the skin. More important, niacin was a cheaply manufactured vitamin that wasn't going to be profitable for any pharmaceutical company. They needed something they could patent.

Since the early days of successful niacin treatment, drug companies have offered patented "no flush" versions—this is actually *niacinamide*, a different thing altogether. The "no flush" version doesn't work in many of the ways that makes straight niacin so effective. The drug makers also came up with a patented "long acting" niacin, but the formulation has a high incidence of liver damage and other toxicities.

The next line of research involved making powders to soak up the bile in the gut and cause cholesterol to be sent out of the body in the stool. These drugs caused bloating, constipation, diarrhea, and excessive gas.

Researchers then turned their attention to seeking a substance that would somehow interrupt the liver's production of cholesterol. They found just such a chemical in certain strains of mold growing on rice. The first medicine made from this mold was named *mevastatin* and since then, all drugs in this class are called *statins.*

The liver uses the nutrients from food as building blocks and goes through ten major steps to pop out cholesterol at the end. A biochemical needed at step one has a particular shape that fits like a key in a lock to speed up the next chemical reaction in the chain—this is called an *enzyme.* Statin drugs have a shape that partially mimics this natural enzyme; a statin acts like an ill-fitting key that blocks the lock. So the body's natural enzyme has to compete with statins to get in there and do its job. In this way, statins slow down the liver's manufacture of cholesterol.

Statins are gradually broken down by other biochemicals in the liver and eventually eliminated in the stool. When a person takes anything else that *also* lowers cholesterol, the statin drugs are more likely to cause side effects. Even today, the mechanisms behind this are not well understood. It can be concluded that if you mess very much with Mother Nature by giving more than one thing to interfere with cholesterol, then you are going to cause a lot of problems.

Statins decrease how much of the LDL type of cholesterol is made in the liver, but may have other indirect effects. A handful of small studies done in humans have suggested particularly high doses of statins may make plaques less inflammatory and may cause some to stop enlarging in a small percentage of patients. There is some evidence to suggest statins decrease the liver's production of irritating proteins, and may slightly and indirectly decrease blood vessel inflammation. Sounds promising! Unfortunately, these effects were only seen in a minority of patients who were on high dose statins. This does not translate into practical use, because most patients are not on the high doses due to the greater incidence of intolerable drug side effects. [1] On the other hand, other studies show exactly the opposite: statin use has been associated with an *accelerated* rate of plaque growth, particularly among diabetics on statins.[2]

All drugs cause some kind of side effects. I think you'll agree: what really proves that a drug is worth its possible side effects is how well it improves quality of life and survival. While statin drugs are associated with a very slight number of decreased deaths from heart disease in select populations, *to what degree will they be helpful to a single individual?* This is the really important part that needs to be explained in the process of full Informed Consent on a patient-by-patient basis.

Just as important, you should know how the statistics on drug effectiveness are reported. The statistics on statin drugs revolve around the rate of illness from *cardiovascular events*, which means heart attacks, heart failure, stroke, and chest pain that cause a need for stent or bypass operation. The drug makers' studies show that when statin drugs are effective at all, they have their most pronounced effect in preventing a cardiovascular event in middle aged men. They are less effective as a person gets older, all the way to the point of being nearly useless in prolonging life in people over 70. [3]

Cardiovascular disease is something that builds up gradually, getting more likely and more severe as we age. So the older we get, the more likely we are to get cardiovascular disease; but as we age, it is less and less likely that statin drugs will do anything to decrease our mortality rate.

Just because statins are effective for some men in middle age does not mean they should be prescribed to everyone. The 'one-size-fits-all' idea promoted by drug advertising is not supported by the evidence. What works in some groups of people may not answer the right question.

Do you need to take a statin drug?

Some people will benefit from being on a statin drug—a very few people— and trying to choose who they will be is the tricky thing. This is in large part because cholesterol alone only contributes *slightly* to cardiovascular risk. It has only a minor role in the drama of cardiovascular disease.

A drug maker sponsored study described in the original package insert for Lipitor showed that 100 people had to take the drug for over three years for one person to avoid a heart attack. How can this be true when the Lipitor ads claimed it reduces heart attacks by 36%? The usual patient who hears this thinks if he takes the drug, he has an impressive 36% less chance of not suffering another heart attack, however, that is not what it means at all.

This impressive-sounding claim came from a study of people who had high cholesterol (250mg/dL or more) and also had several additional risk factors for heart disease. Over the course of three and half years, those taking Lipitor were compared to those taking only a sugar pill (placebo). Among every 100 people, 3 people on placebo had a heart attack and 2 people on Lipitor had heart attacks. The '2' versus the '3' is where the "approximately 36%" claim mentioned in the package insert and on TV commercials comes from. But as you can see from the simple math, only 1 heart attack in 100 people over three and a half years can be blamed on lack of Lipitor. [4]

Let's say we equate persons at risk for a heart attack to old cars at risk for tire blowouts. When 100 clunkers are continuously driven for three and a half years on generic tires, three blowouts are expected to occur. 100 cars with "Lipitires" could be driven for three and a half years with only two blowouts happening. The reduction from 3 down to 2 blowouts equates to approximately one third fewer blowouts. It also means that 99 out of 100 not rolling on the special tires are not at any increased risk, despite using generic tires. Riding on Lipitires has no substantial benefit—they are nearly as likely to experience a blowout as those on the usual tires. Nevertheless, the Lipitire commercials can truthfully claim a one-third reduction in blowouts because they've determined which math to highlight. Why would they do this? To improve marketability. Always keep in mind that a drug company is a company established and managed to the same goal as any other company: to generate profit margins.

What the study numbers actually mean is that *two out of every one hundred were going to have a heart attack anyway*. The one more heart attack per hundred occurring in the placebo group was blamed on a lack of Lipitor. It took 100 people to take Lipitor for three and a half years in order to prevent one heart attack, 97 of them were never going to have a heart attack anyway, and 2 were going to have heart attacks even if they took Lipitor. A useful way of looking at the prediction of any one individual having a benefit from a drug is to consider the number-needed-to-treat in order to prevent a cardiovascular event. In this study, 100 is designated as the number-needed-to-treat: in other words, 100 high-risk people had to take the drug for over three years in order for 1 heart attack to be avoided in 1 person.

Of course, the drug maker wants everyone to be on statin drugs, not just high-risk people. If this statistical analysis were extended beyond just the people with high risk for a heart attack to the general adult population, then the number-needed-to-treat would be more like 250 to 500. The number-needed–to-treat is much more meaningful to an individual patient than are the relative risk reduction statistics.

Do you presume that your doctor has done some special test to determine you are the 1 in 100 who should take the drug?

Sorry, there is no test to identify that *one* who would be most likely to benefit. These statistics paint a very different story than the TV commercials. What is good for a few is not best for all.

At the time of the Lipitor study, the cost of the drug was over $1,400 per year. That added up to $3,959,501 spent on Lipitor prescriptions with no benefit in 99 people over the course of three and a half years. All patients were at risk for drug-induced muscle damage, increased cancer incidence, and possible premature dementia among numerous other side effects. In 1 out of 100 it may have been worth the side effects in order to prevent a heart attack, but the other 99 suffered side effects only, with no benefit from the drug at all.

CHAPTER 6

UNDERSTANDING CHOLESTEROL NUMBERS

Americans have been urged to get their cholesterol numbers checked and be watchful of the magic number calling for drug treatment. In this chapter, you will learn about routine cholesterol testing and what triggers drug treatment.

Cholesterol is not represented by just one number. This is because the total cholesterol circulating in the blood is the sum of many different particles of varying sizes and densities, or compactness. Cholesterol circulates as *lipoproteins:* one part protein and one part fat.

A routine blood test includes Total Cholesterol, Low Density Lipoproteins, High Density Lipoproteins, and Triglycerides. The usual measurement is given as milligrams per one-tenth liter of blood (mg/dL), but the units will be left off for the purposes of this discussion. When statin drugs first came on the market, cholesterol-lowering medicines were only recommended for people with multiple risk factors for heart disease who also had total cholesterol over 250.

The high-density lipoproteins, HDL, are smaller and denser. HDL is the form of cholesterol moving out of circulation and getting deposited into the liver where it gets removed or recycled. HDL is protective against heart disease: the higher this number, the better.

The basic cholesterol report often includes a risk ratio: Total cholesterol (TC) divided by the amount of high density lipoproteins (TC/HDL). A lower number means less risk of heart disease. In other words, the greater proportion of total cholesterol that is the high-density kind (HDL) the better. The American Heart Association suggests the goal is a ratio of 5 to 1 or lower. A low Total/HDL ratio assures at least one fifth of the total circulating cholesterol is the good HDL kind.

The low-density lipoproteins, LDL, are larger and less compact, contain more cholesterol, and have been identified as a risk factor in the development of heart disease. However, many people with heart attacks don't have high LDL levels, and many people with high LDL levels never get a heart attack. This means LDL is only a *minor* risk factor in *some* people. In other people, LDL does not appear to pose any risk at all. It is necessary to take a closer look at the back story of the cholesterol mania to understand why this minor player has gotten so much attention—why LDL is the focus of recommendations to take medication and why the TV ads scare you about your LDL level.

In 1988, the National Cholesterol Education Program (NCEP) set itself up as an authority on cholesterol levels. That year, the Adult Treatment Panel of the NCEP published recommendations for who should get treatment with statins, and when. Because of all of the conflicting medical literature on the effectiveness of statins and their adverse effects, the panelists essentially *voted* on what to recommend. The first NCEP Adult Treatment recommendations in 1988 advised statin therapy for anyone who had an LDL at or above 160, or LDL at 130 if the person had two or more additional risk factors. That made about 13 million Americans eligible for statin drugs overnight, by vote. [1]

The next update came from NCEP in 1993 and said the optimal LDL should be less than 130 for everybody, including women and young adults. The 1993 recommendations urged regular cholesterol testing for all Americans starting at age 20. This made hundreds of thousands more Americans eligible for statin drugs.

What's even more interesting is that all but one of the panelists was or had been in the pay of various manufacturers or distributors of cholesterol lowering drugs. [2]

A crucial aspect of informed consent is to consider conflicts of interest and their influence on drug recommendations. In this case, it is easy to follow the money: the experts were laden with drug company ties and kept lowering the "acceptable" cholesterol levels, which increased their target market. People who used to be considered "normal" were moved to the "too high" category, creating more people to sell drugs to.

A third set of Adult Treatment recommendations came in 2001. A major change in this version was to consider diabetes and various non-heart vascular conditions as "equivalents to cardiovascular disease." These included narrowing of the arteries in the legs or neck and weakening of the wall of the large vessel in the abdomen (aortic aneurysm). The main message of the 2001 guidelines was that the new optimal goal was to achieve an LDL under 100. Even though the guidelines only recommended this degree of lowering for people in the highest risk group who already had heart disease or an equivalent, it became common practice to target an LDL of 100 or less with statin therapy for *everyone*. Upon publishing these recommendations, the NCEP predicted their new guidelines would triple the number of Americans on statins from 13 million to 36 million. [3]

Cha-ching for the pharmaceutical company stockholders!

By 2001 there were more requirements in place to disclose conflicts of interest than there were back in 1988 and 1993. The 2001 nine-person panel included only one who did not have any potential conflicts to report. The remaining eight received funding in one form or another from all of the major manufacturers or distributors of cholesterol-lowering drugs and other pharma companies. The disclosures were posted on the website of the NCEP's government sponsor, the National Heart Lung and Blood Institute (NHLBI)—at least they were there through December of 2014. Despite the NHLBI's commitment to transparency, the link to the disclosures is no longer working. The full list can still be accessed elsewhere.[4] The list is too impressive to summarize, so here it is in full:

Dr. Grundy: received honoraria from Merck, Pfizer, Sankyo, Bayer, Bristol-Myers Squibb, and AstraZeneca; he has received research grants from Merck, Abbott, and Glaxo Smith Kline.

Dr. Bairey Merz: received lecture honoraria from Pfizer, Merck, and Kos; she has served as a consultant for Pfizer, Bayer, and EHC

(Merck); has received unrestricted institutional grants for Continuing Medical Education from Pfizer, Procter & Gamble, Novartis, Wyeth, AstraZeneca, and Bristol-Myers Squibb Medical Imaging; has received a research grant from Merck; has stock in Boston Scientific, IVAX, Eli Lilly, Medtronic, Johnson & Johnson, SCIPIE Insurance, ATS Medical, and Biosite.

Dr. Brewer: received honoraria from AstraZeneca, Pfizer, Lipid Sciences, Merck, Merck/Schering-Plough, Fournier, Tularik, Esperion, and Novartis; he has served as a consultant for AstraZeneca, Pfizer, Lipid Sciences, Merck, Merck/Schering-Plough, Fournier, Tularik, Sankyo, and Novartis.

Dr. Clark: received honoraria for educational presentations from Abbott, AstraZeneca, Bristol-Myers Squibb, Merck, and Pfizer; he has received grant/research support from Abbott, AstraZeneca, Bristol-Myers Squibb, Merck, and Pfizer.

Dr. Hunninghake: received honoraria for consulting and speakers bureau from AstraZeneca, Merck, Merck/Schering-Plough, and Pfizer, and for consulting from Kos; he has received research grants from AstraZeneca, Bristol-Myers Squibb, Kos, Merck, Merck/Schering-Plough, Novartis, and Pfizer.

Dr. Pasternak: served as a paid speaker for Pfizer, Merck, Merck/Schering-Plough, Takeda, Kos, BMS-Sanofi, and Novartis; he has served as a consultant for Merck, Merck/Schering-Plough, Sanofi, Pfizer Health Solutions, Johnson & Johnson-Merck, and AstraZeneca.

Dr. Smith: received institutional research support from Merck; he has stock in Medtronic and Johnson & Johnson.

Dr. Stone: received honoraria for educational lectures from Abbott, AstraZeneca, Bristol-Myers Squibb, Kos, Merck, Merck/Schering-Plough, Novartis, Pfizer, Reliant, and Sankyo; he has served as a consultant for Abbott, Merck, Merck/Schering-Plough, Pfizer, and Reliant.

You don't have to be a conspiracy theorist to see what is wrong with allowing people who are in the pocket of the drug makers to establish drug treatment guidelines. That is something like making your dog in charge of the Committee to Distribute Doggie Treats.

In 2004, the recommendations were updated further, pushing the treatment goal down again to LDL of less than 70 for some patients. [5] This was all going on while more data was piling up from studies showing that lowering LDL was not the right target. In the meantime, cholesterol-lowering drugs became the number one star of all stars in the entire history of drugs sales.

Since then, a variety of other expert panels have jostled for their own guidelines to take precedence. A review of the conflicts of interest amongst authors of various cholesterol guidelines was conducted in 2011. It was found that out of 14 guidelines published, more than a third didn't report the author's conflicts of interest at all. Out of the remaining 288 panel members, 138 (almost half) reported conflicts of interest at the time of the guideline publication, but no information on earlier financial relationships that may have influenced the results. 73 panelists formally declared no conflicts, but 8 of them (11%) were later found to have undisclosed conflicts. This brought the total with known conflicts to 52%, again with more than a third not even reporting. [6]

Just for perspective, if your investment advisor didn't disclose his conflicts, he would probably be disbarred from working in the financial advisory world ever again. Why is it ok for these medical experts to get away with it?

In 2013, the American Heart Association and the American College of Cardiology jointly published yet another set of cholesterol guidelines. They combined the LDL level with various patient characteristics into classifications for statin treatment. In short, they recommend high-intensity statin therapy for anyone up to age 76, for anyone with cardiovascular disease, and for anyone with LDL 190 or above, and for certain high-risk diabetics. Moderate inensity therapy is advised for just about anyone else with LDL over 70. These guidelines effectively endorsed the acceptable LDL to 70 for nearly everyone.

In the American Heart Association/American Association of Cardiology Cholesterol Guidelines article, fully seven pages of an appendix lists the potential conflicts of interest of the authors. About half of the panelists listed potential conflicts with makers of cholesterol lowering drugs, and the most frequently paying companies were Merck (maker of Mevacor, Zocor, Zetia, Vytorin, Liptruzet) and Pfizer (maker of Lipitor). [7]

If lowering cholesterol helps prevent heart attacks, does it matter who is paying the guideline authors? That question calls for a closer scrutiny of the studies concluding statin drugs are effective at all.

CHAPTER 7

DO STATINS WORK?

About one-third of heart attack victims have normal LDL levels, and nearly all Americans who experience a second heart attack are already on a statin drug. In other words, LDL cholesterol is not a heart risk factor for many people, and for others it may be a *minor* risk factor.

How did the statins get to be blockbuster drugs with statistics like that?

Four landmark studies published in rapid succession in a five-year period were the key to promoting aggressive use of statin drugs. All of the studies were done on high-risk patients (those with known existing cardiovascular disease or, in one study, diabetes). These are not your everyday patients who have relatively minor family history and/or LDL levels above 100. They were all funded through manufacturer-sponsored foundations or grants from statin manufacturers or distributors. Here are the outcomes and weaknesses to the studies.

LIPID Trial

(Long Term Intervention with Pravastatin in Ischemic Disease) [1998]

This study made the sponsor's drug Pravachol (pravastatin) look spectacular, but repeat studies did not bear the same fabulous results. There are serious flaws in the study design and some of the statistics reported are inexplicable—they don't make any kind of medical sense. The LIPID trial, sponsored by Bristol-Myers Squibb, was one of the most impressive early mega-studies to follow patients on statins for five years or more. About 4,500 high-risk people with a history of unstable angina or heart attack were given pravastatin and about an equal number were given placebo. The authors calculated that there were highly significant reductions in death due to heart disease and vascular disease in the pravastatin group, and they calculated reduced hospitalizations for strokes, stents, or angina. The authors concluded, "…the current low rate of use of cholesterol-lowering therapy among patients with CHD [coronary heart disease] can no longer be accepted." This implied that any doctor who failed to aggressively prescribe statin drugs to high-risk patients was threatening the health and life of his patients. [1]

Even though this study focused exclusively on high-risk patients who had already experienced a heart attack or unstable angina, the author's strong conclusions were used to rocket the worldwide popularity of statins for everyone, regardless of not having risk factors. It served to promote statin sales into blockbuster status. But subsequent studies on the same drug, in a similar high-risk population, *were not shown to have the same effect.* This makes the spectacular LIPID study results highly suspect when they could not be reproduced in other studies. Studies have also failed to show much, *if any,* benefit in people who never had a heart attack or unstable angina. The take-home point is that the study was never designed to look at people who have high cholesterol and no heart attack or chest pain. If that is you, or it sounds like someone you know, keep in mind that even the weak results of this study do not apply to you.

The statistics were calculated to give impressive results in this pravastatin study, but they came into question because of the wide variances in medication use. By the end of the study, some of the pravastatin group were also on other cholesterol lowering medications, and nearly a fifth of the patients on pravastatin had in fact stopped taking the drug. To make matters even more confusing, nearly a quarter of the patients in the placebo group were being prescribed other cholesterol-lowering drugs, including statins. How could the researchers make sense of the numbers when the comparison groups were so varied? Aside from muddying the waters to find any drug benefit, the mixed nature of the groups *totally invalidated* the comparison of adverse drug effects. There were many people taking some cholesterol lowering drug or other in the so-called placebo group, so how could you credibly rate side effects compared to placebo? Scientifically, this is impossible!

PROSPER Study

(Prospective Study of Pravastatin in the Elderly at Risk) [2002]

This was another large study on pravastatin and this one showed much less benefit in the elderly than had been seen in younger people. The PROSPER study was also sponsored by Bristol-Myers Squibb. The subjects consisted of more than 5,800 patients, age 70 and older, with either a history of vascular disease or cardiovascular risk factors. About half took the drug, half took placebo.

Coming only a few years after the LIPID study, this study failed to reproduce the same results in the people taking the drug. The participants did achieve lower LDL levels, but there was *no difference* in the percentage that died compared to those taking only a sugar pill (placebo). There were not significantly fewer angioplasties or bypasses, nor were there significantly fewer hospital admissions for heart failure in those on pravastatin. In the pravastatin group, there were fewer cardiovascular events (which included coronary heart disease death, heart attacks, and strokes), however, this advantage was only *2.1 percentage points.*

Most importantly, it did not translate into improved survival since all-cause death (death from any cause) was the same as in the group that took only placebo. In other words, individuals in both groups died at the same rate, so there was no survival advantage to taking the drug. In fact, the most significant finding of this study was the whopping 25% increase in cancer diagnoses in the pravastatin treated group. [2]

The PROSPER study was also designed to test if pravastatin would reduce the incidence of stroke or slow the development of dementia in the elderly (ages 70-82 years). The rates of stroke and dementia were not statistically different among those on pravastatin compared to those on placebo.

Yet the paper concluded with an endorsement of applying the same statin treatment guidelines used for middle-aged people to statin treatment in the elderly. These marginal results would not logically lead to such a sweeping conclusion. A more reasonable conclusion would have been to voice extreme caution about translating the results of the LIPID study (which looked at pravastatin use in middle age) to long-term use of the drugs well into the older age group.

Clearly, this study showed any slight benefit at a younger age tended to disappear as a person gets older. The fact that the sweeping conclusion is so opposite to the actual study results raises a suspicion of conflict of interest. Sure enough, twenty three of the study authors, including the three lead researchers, disclosed paid consultancy agreements or had received research support, travel grants, and/or other paid benefits from the study sponsor or other statin manufacturers.

MIRACL Trial

(Myocardial Ischemia Reduction with Acute Cholesterol Lowering) [2002]

This is another study where the dismal results did not justify the authors' resounding conclusions endorsing widespread statin use. In the MIRACL study funded by Pfizer, patients who had suffered a heart attack were immediately given high dose atorvastatin for 16 weeks. The study did not show a statistically significant reduction in a recurrent heart attack, death, or cardiac arrest. Nevertheless, the authors concluded that high dose atorvastatin would be beneficial to give in the immediate post-heart attack period. [3]

Why would they write such a pro-drug conclusion?

You guessed it: six of the ten lead authors were or had been the beneficiary of research funding, consultancy fees, speakers fees, lecture fees, or expense reimbursement from Pfizer or other drug makers.

HPS Study

(Heart Protection Study) [2003]

This was another pharma-funded study that used deceptively impressive *"relative"* statistical analysis to cover the fact that the *absolute* reduction in heart attack deaths was ridiculously small. HPS was a Merck-funded study of their drug simvastatin in high-risk patients. All persons in the study had existing heart disease, hardening of the arteries, and/or diabetes. Over 10,000 people were put on simvastatin and compared to about an equal number on placebo over a five year period.

After five years, results showed 12.9% of those on simvastatin had died while 14.7% of those on placebo had died, for an *Absolute Risk Reduction* of 1.8 percentage points. A subset of the deaths was the coronary death rate: 5.7% in those on the drug versus 6.9% in those on placebo for a difference of 1.2 percentage points.

Another way of looking at the same numbers is to see that the heart related deaths killed 0.73% of all the people on simvastatin and similarly killed 1.0% of all of the people who were not on simvastatin. This amounts to a difference of about one-quarter of one percentage point— small indeed. So, 400 people who already had one heart attack would have to take this drug for 5 years for just 1 person to avoid another heart attack. Considering the potential side effects of statin drugs, these are not impressive numbers even for people who already had a heart attack. The number-needed-to-treat for one person to benefit would be much greater than 400 among people that don't fall into the 'already had a heart attack' category.

In this study, like many others, some of the patients in both groups were also on other heart medications, including other statin drugs besides simvastatin. This makes it a very poorly controlled study and invalidates any assessment of comparative rates of drug side effects. [4]

JUPITER Trial

At this time, the majority of people on statins are not in a high-risk group despite the efforts to broaden the definition of "risk." Studies focusing on high-risk patients cannot necessarily be applied to people who don't have clinically important heart or vascular disease. Here is a summary of the largest of these, the JUPITER trial (Justification for the Use of Statins in Primary Prevention: An Intervention Trial Evaluating Rosuvastatin). This study has been highly criticized in the professional medical world as a flagrant example of excessive pharma-sponsored influence on study conduct.

JUPITER was funded by AstraZeneca, maker of rosuvastatin. The 17,802 patients in this study did not have heart disease, and their LDL levels were normal or low. They were selected because they had elevated levels of C-reactive protein (CRP). CRP is an inflammatory marker not specific to heart disease, but is an indicator of the risk of developing heart disease, heart attack, or sudden death.

Half of the subjects were given rosuvastatin and half were given a placebo. The median duration of follow up was only 1.9 years. At that point, the study was stopped because the researchers felt they had achieved a significant result, namely that rosuvastatin-treated subjects had a lower rate of major cardiovascular events. Astra-Zeneca stock soared upon publication of the results. However, doctors were not keen to embrace the results and did not change their prescribing habits as stockholders had hoped.

Immediate criticisms of the JUPITER study included scrutiny of some odd statistics: there were significant reductions in *nonfatal* strokes and heart attacks, but no fewer fatal strokes or fatal heart attacks. This is called "clinically inconsistent": it was not what was expected and there was no explanation for it.

By the time the trial was concluded, the benefits to the drug group were getting ever smaller. This has led to speculation that if the trial had been continued even a little bit longer, the differences seen initially between the drug group and the placebo would have become minimal. The trial was stopped just as the drug was showing benefit, but the results at 1.9 years probably would have washed out within just one more year.

The JUPITER study also revealed how many people would have to take the drug for one person to benefit. The number needed to treat with rosuvastatin to prevent one cardiovascular event was 95 over a period of two years. That means 95 healthy people would be taking the drug daily for two years to prevent 1 cardiovascular event in 1 person. [5]

There have been suspicions voiced that AstraZeneca may have had too much to do with the study design and results. Nine of fourteen authors of the JUPITER study had financial relationships directly with AstraZeneca. The study's lead researcher also holds a patent interest in the specific test used to measure C-reactive protein (CRP), a general indicator of body inflammation. All of this adds up to a useless study only beneficial for a short-term stock jump.

Making Sense of the Statin Studies

A unique group of physicians and statisticians performed their own rigorous analysis of statin studies. They specifically looked at the concept of number-needed-to-treat (NNT). Their summaries can be found on NNT.com. This is a web-published group consisting of doctors who evaluate therapies "based on their patient-important benefits and harms." Most notably, they accept no outside funding or advertisements.

The NNT analysis combined the JUPITER results with a number of other studies of statin use in people who were not in a high-risk category. Here's how all these studies break down and what that means for you:

It was found that although statins do lower cholesterol in most people, very few people avoid a heart attack or stroke, and death rates are not affected at all. This underscores that cholesterol is only a weak risk factor, if it is a risk factor at all. The average individual would have to take statins for five years to have a shot at a 1.6% chance of avoiding heart attack and a 0.37% chance of avoiding a stroke. When statins are taken over that duration, diabetes or muscle damage is easier to get than avoiding a heart attack; 1 in 50 would develop diabetes from the drugs, and 1 in 10 would get painful and possibly permanent muscle damage. [6]

If you look across the entire US population, avoiding one heart death out of a few hundred is quite a lot. But to the guy who asks his doctor, "Is this drug worthwhile for *me* to take?" the national statistics simply don't apply, especially considering the drug side effects. No fully informed decision about taking statins can be made without taking a look at the possible downside of the drugs.

CHAPTER 8

CHOLESTEROL AND YOUR BRAIN

Statin makers want everyone on their drugs, even those without particular risk factors for heart disease. There are plenty of doctors who are on this bandwagon, totally willing to ignore the most fundamental principle of 'first do no harm' or simply relying foolishly on packaging from the manufacturer instead of looking any futher to make that judgement themselves.

The body has evolved over hundreds of generations to operate as an incredibly complex web of interdependent systems. Early on in pharmaceutical history there was a popular myth of the magic bullet that would bring about a miraculous cure, but otherwise leave no trace. It is a fact that a pharmaceutical approach to the human body never affects only one specific area or an isolated biochemical activity.

Nothing like a magic bullet exists in a prescription drug.

That is why the term 'side effects' has been abandoned and replaced with the more accurate phrase 'adverse drug effects.' In other words, there are good effects we want and bad effects we didn't intend to happen. The more widespread the drug's target, the more likely there will be serious adverse drug effects. Today's drugs can be more like shooting a cannon ball into a church tower to kill one sniper and, unfortunately, also bringing the roof crashing down on the whole innocent congregation.

In the case of statin drugs, interfering with the body's natural cholesterol metabolism in order to reduce heart attacks also deranges cholesterol's role in many other body functions. Cholesterol is the building block for sex hormones (testosterone, estrogen, and progesterone) and for cortisol, the hormone we use to respond to stress; the main component of bile, which assures we can absorb vitamins A, D, E, and K; and a basic component of cell membranes, where it facilitates communication among cells so your body functions as a live being rather than a lump of unrelated cells.

Between the year 2000 and 2010, the number of deaths from heart disease went down by 16%, largely attributed by statin manufacturers to widespread use of statin drugs. As we've already seen in earlier chapters, it is highly unlikely the improvement was due to statin use. However, in the same ten years, the number of deaths from Alzheimer's dementia rose by 68%. Is there a correlation? [1]

It is logical to assume that if people are not dying from heart attacks at a younger age, they live long enough to get dementia in old age. But, it actually doesn't work out like that. In the two decades from 1990-2010, the cardiovascular *age-adjusted death rate*[2] went down by 43% and was almost mirrored by a 39% increase in the *age-adjusted death rate* from Alzheimer's. [3] It wasn't that people who escaped heart attack deaths lived long enough to eventually get Alzheimer's. Rather, it means the same age people who are avoiding heart deaths are instead dying from dementia.

While it is alarming to be taken out quickly by a heart attack, most people would agree it is almost more worrisome to think about deteriorating slowly with the confusion and memory loss of dementia. To understand how cholesterol comes into the picture, it is necessary to understand that *brain cholesterol has an entirely different story than blood cholesterol*. We know that cholesterol is a building block for every single cell in the body, but it is important to also know it is vitally important to proper brain functioning in particular. You need to take all the information you've been told about how bad cholesterol is and be willing to look at it in another light.

The basic science of brain biochemistry supports the notion that statins may cause increased dementia. The brain accounts for only 2% of the body's mass, but contains a quarter of the body's total cholesterol. Cholesterol in the brain facilitates the speed of nerve transmission, promotes the fighting of infection, and protects against damaging biochemical reactions that would promote cancer. "If you deprive cholesterol from the brain, then you directly affect the machinery responsible for triggering the release of neurotransmitters. Neurotransmitters affect data processing and memory functions. In other words — how smart you are and how well you remember things," says a leading cholesterol researcher at Iowa State University. [4]

When non-demented people age 85 to 101 were given memory tests, researchers at Mount Sinai School of Medicine proved that those with the highest LDL and highest overall total cholesterol were those with the best memory scores. People with higher cholesterol have better memories. [5]

The fact that higher cholesterol in old age is associated with less chance of dementia was also shown by researchers from Johns Hopkins University. They evaluated the records of elderly people and found that increased cholesterol levels, when measured at the age of 70, were associated with a reduced risk of dementia when those same people were between the ages of 79 and 88. [6]

Most of the brain's cholesterol is found in the outer coating of *neurons* (brain cells) that transmit nerve signals. This coating is called *myelin* and it acts like insulation, magnifying the travelling speed of the nerve signals to almost 400 feet per second. Without myelin, nerve impulses would travel sluggishly and as a result the brain (and body) would not work too well.

The brain of a fetus starts to lay its miles of myelin at 14-weeks; this goes into high production during infancy and continues into the teen years. That is why babies and children need relatively higher-fat diets than adults. So, you can see cholesterol is very important to normal brain development.

Some cholesterol is cranked out in the brain's star-shaped cells—the so-called *astrocytes* (astro – "star" + – cytes "cells")—and this continues at a low level in adults. The cholesterol made in astrocytes has extremely important functions in the brain. It helps form communication bridges between nerve endings, stimulates the long branching brain cells to grow longer, and protects against brain cell death. In fact, anytime there is a brain injury, the astrocytes amp up cholesterol production by 150 times over normal in order to repair the damage. Cholesterol is very important to proper brain function throughout every phase of human life.

The body has a built-in mechanism to protect the brain called the blood-brain barrier. This barrier prevents most toxins (and many drugs) from penetrating the brain, but it turns out statin drugs can get through that barrier. Lovastatin and simvastatin are the best at this, followed by atorvastatin, fluvastatin, and rosuvastatin; pravastatin is the poorest at penetrating into the brain. When these drugs get into the brain, they go to work blocking cholesterol production.

We know one of the roles of brain cholesterol is to facilitate the millions of communication connections between brain cells. Statins crossing into the brain are interfering with production of this valuable cholesterol, and not much is known about how the brain might have a means to overcome this effect.

The natural enzyme coQ10 is part of the cholesterol biochemical pathways. CoQ10 is protective to brain cells and plays a role in healthy aging and prevention of dementia. The statin drugs not only decrease cholesterol, but they also profoundly diminish the levels of natural enzyme coQ10.

The body's normal cholesterol production cannot be manipulated without also affecting other processes reliant upon the same mechanisms. Studies on the effects of statins on mice brains have demonstrated that long-term treatment with atorvastatin causes changes in brain biochemistry. This results in behavioral deficits (treated mice didn't play well in an open field) and intelligence (treated mice were less successful reaching the cheese at the end of a maze). Mice metabolize cholesterol similar to the way humans do, so the mouse model is predictive of the effects these drugs would have in humans. [7]

Patients and their physicians have submitted hundreds of reports of statin drugs causing memory loss and confusion. Some of these occurred after just one day on the drug. A well-publicized instance of this was described in a book by the victim, himself a physician. When Duane Graveline, MD—a former NASA astronaut and aerospace physician—was put on Lipitor, he had a prolonged spell of disordered thinking, completely loosing his short-term memory. He simply could not retain any new things he was experiencing or learning. He stopped the drug and his symptoms resolved, but no one was sure it was a drug effect. The following year, he resumed Lipitor at half dose and lost both short-term memory and memories from long ago. When he showed up in such a state in an emergency room, he was diagnosed with amnesia. The memory loss was short lived (transient) and affected all memory domains (global). [8] *Transient Global Amnesia* is now listed on the package insert as an adverse drug effect. [9]

Briefer moments of memory loss and confusion also occur while on statins, but are much less likely to be reported because they are more often chalked up to the result of normal aging, "senior moments." Some studies have demonstrated that those on statins score worse on cognitive tests. Dr. Graveline estimates that statins are causing short episodes of memory loss every day, but too few are suspecting their medication may be the culprit. Just as coQ10 reduces the impact of aging throughout the body, it also does so in the brain. Drastically reduced levels of coQ10 and cholesterol caused by statin drugs may result in damage that cannot be undone. [10]

Vitamin D is made naturally by the sun triggering a reaction in the skin, which rearranges the molecular position of cholesterol in the skin. The result is vitamin D: a molecule that looks almost exactly like cholesterol. People on statin drugs also tend to have reduced levels of vitamin D. Low vitamin D is associated with heart disease, life threatening infections, increased risk of some cancers, bone disease, and most importantly, improper brain development and function. [11]

You may have heard news reports that statin drugs may prevent Alzheimer's dementia. How can that be when the same drugs may cause memory loss and confusion, and people with high cholesterol have better memories, lower risk of dementia, and live longer? Is this simply another sketchy claim made by researchers who have conflicts of interest? Or, just advertising cooked up by the pharmaceutical company? Let's look at the real science.

There is a current theory that the key to aging is *inflammation*: damage from various toxins or other insults to the body provoke inflammation. The cumulative effects of chronic inflammation finally overwhelm a body system. It is possible that disease (such as diabetes, heart attack, stroke, or dementia) is the long-term result of ongoing inflammation. Alzheimer's dementia may be caused by the brain's response to chronic inflammation in susceptible people.

Some years ago it was noticed that aside from lowering cholesterol, statin drugs also have mild anti-inflammatory properties. That is, they quiet down and may even prevent inflammation. This is the theory underlying the idea that statins may help prevent Alzheimer's. It is possible that the slight positive effects of statins on reducing heart attack and stroke in younger patients with high risks are *more from their anti-inflammatory effects than from lowering cholesterol*. Cholesterol-lowering may be an incidental effect, and we may have been barking up the wrong tree all along.

The risk for the Alzheimer kind of dementia seems to hinge to some extent on what kind of cholesterol a person makes, and which kind depends on inherited genes. People who have the APOE4 gene have the highest risk of getting old-age Alzheimer's dementia. Only 15% of the population has this gene and not all of them get dementia; they are just more likely to get it. It is thought that the APOE4 gene has something to do with poorly operating cholesterol transportation. Brain cholesterol is just not well regulated in some people with the APOE4 genes. So it was logical to suspect that maybe giving brain-penetrating cholesterol-lowering statin drugs could prevent dementia, but it has not been proven in tests. Drug makers were hoping statins would prevent or reverse the consequences of brain inflammation, and this in turn may prevent Alzheimer's dementia. Two large studies funded by drug companies failed to show their drugs (pravastatin and atorvastatin) did anything to prevent Alzheimer's.

In a 2005 study looking at the health records of a large Health Maintenance Organization, statin treatment of people with any cholesterol type was initially reported as being significantly protective against the development of dementia. However, in a subsequent analysis of the same data, the researchers confessed that they manipulated the data to show a favorable result; they later said it was not a valid way to look at the numbers as it only gave the false impression of a benefit not really there. [12] This was just one more example of misleading reporting based on faulty statistical analysis. How many people were prescribed statins unneccessarily because of the misleading initial report? How many doctors bothered to read the second analysis?

In a 2007 study, researchers scrutinized a large Veteran's Administration database and found veterans taking simvastatin had only half the incidence of Alzheimer's compared with those not on any statin drug. *However, it is important to note that no subsequent study has been able to reproduce these results.* It is very likely that bias entered into this study and that everything else going on with those patients was not taken into consideration. What other meds were they taking, were they more likely to exercise, or was there some other common characteristic that protected against Alzheimer's? When such things are unknown, then they may be biasing the results. In an attempt to validate whether their findings meant simvastatin reduces Alzheimer's, the researchers conducted autopsies. Brains of patients on simvastatin did not show any fewer globs of Alzheimer's-associated proteins. This makes the entire study inconclusive.

Oh, one more thing: the study's lead researcher held a patent for use of statin as therapy for Alzheimer's disease. [13]

When people with the APOE4 gene are put on statin drugs, it generally lowers their cholesterol levels in the blood. But, it is not known what is happening to cholesterol levels in the brain because we don't have a good way to measure this without getting into the brain somehow. And that's just messy. Some studies showed those on statins had less chance of getting dementia, *some showed an increased risk of dementia on statins*, and other studies showed no change either way. How could there be differing results from studies of the same drugs? As we have seen, poor study design and statistical manipulation can give you pretty much any answer you want.

To sort this out, an international medical review group looked at *all* statin dementia studies. They could only identify four studies that met their criteria of being *randomized* (patients were randomly selected to be given either placebo or drug) and *double blind* (neither researcher nor patient knew at the time if they were on placebo or drug). The end result? The combined numbers did not show any protective effect of statins on preventing dementia. [14]

In another study, the health of nearly 1,000 elderly nuns and priests were followed for 12 years. Unlike the earlier VA study, the ones in this study who had been on statin drugs were no less likely to develop Alzheimer's than people who were not on statins. [15]

In addition to statins possibly harming the brain in terms of memory and cognition, there is a concern that manipulation of cholesterol levels could lead to other disturbances. There are a number of large, well-done studies that have demonstrated adults of any age with naturally low levels of total cholesterol, LDL, or triglycerides have a *greater* chance of depression, suicidal thoughts, and suicide attempts. [16, 17]

While headlines will continue to scream "Statins May Prevent Alzheimer's" from time to time, science *does not* support recommending statins for Alzheimer's dementia prevention or treatment. It wasn't until 2012 that the FDA was moved to instruct statin manufacturers to beef up their mandatory warnings about memory loss and confusion. But they are only required to list these possible adverse effects as "mild" and "temporary." It is not likely any individual considers his own drug-induced confusion and memory loss to be trivial—it is downright scary to face the prospect of losing one's mind.

The mandatory warnings about memory deficits did not curb the broad dissemination of the results of a study e-published in December 2016, which links high dose statin use to reduced risk of dementia. [18] This was extremely misrepresented in the media, but it is not what it seems.

In the new study, number-crunchers analyzed insurance claims of almost 400,000 patients who were on statin drugs. Notice that they did not compare this group to people not taking a statin. Instead, they took note of the dose of statin each person was on and divided them into a high dose group and a low dose group. They found that for two of the drugs, in some racial and sex groups, people on the high doses developed dementia at a lower rate than the ones on a low dose.

This was widely reported as if statin drugs prevent dementia. What it actually shows is that at high doses, *some* of the statins are *less likely* to cause dementia than at low doses.

The fact is that previous reports amply document the harmful effects of statins on thinking and memory. The FDA has progressively increased mandatory warnings on the prescription insert for this class of drugs. Here are a couple of cases recently reported in the Journal of Medical Case Reports [19] (redacted for brevity):

"Our first patient was a 32-year-old…. He complained of forgetfulness resulting in significant losses to his business one month after initiation of simvastatin. He had impaired recall and memory. He did not complain of any disturbances in his memory prior to starting simvastatin, despite being known to the services for several years. The collateral history from his family confirmed that there had been significant, noticeable impairment related to short-term memory that led him to forget some major business transactions he had carried out. History from our patient and his family was obtained to rule out any possible contributory factors for his symptoms. Our patient did not have any family history of hypercholesterolemia. He had no features to suggest any vascular events in the preceding months that may have contributed to the fairly rapid development of cognitive dysfunction. Our patient had been stable in his mental state for more than 1 year at the time he developed cognitive symptoms. His memory, as reported by our patient as well as his relatives, improved significantly after simvastatin was stopped."

"Our second patient was a 54-year-old... She developed memory impairment and difficulty executing day-to-day activities 2 months after starting simvastatin... As in the case of our first patient, there were no prior complaints of memory symptoms. Her history was obtained from her husband to rule out other possible causes for her symptoms... Her mental state had been stable for several years prior to the development of cognitive symptoms. She did not have any neurological abnormalities on examination and her MRI was normal. No abnormalities were noted in biochemical testing, including her lipid profile... On initial testing, there was impairment in the domains of recall, attention, visual construction, memory, executive functions, and language, which improved after discontinuation of simvastatin."

If statins are indeed toxic to the brain, then wouldn't higher doses be even more toxic? Although most poisons do work that way, there are plenty of exceptions, including some hormones, metals, pesticides, herbicides, and plastic byproducts, to name a few. [20] For example:

- At low doses, tamoxifen stimulates breast cancer growth. At higher does, it inhibits it.

- Bisphenol-A (found in plastic bottles, pool toys, and inflatable balls) causes large tumors to grow at moderate doses, but at high doses that effect goes away.

- The pesticide atrazine causes throat constriction at low doses, but not at high doses.

- In treating early stage breast cancer, a shorter course of radiation therapy at higher doses is less toxic than a longer course at lower doses.

These are all examples of a so-called non-monotonic response, where the lower dose is more toxic than the higher dose.

Again, the recent study on statins only compared people on low dose statins to people on high dose statins. There was no comparison to people not on statins at all. Such studies have been done. Some have shown no effect on preventing dementia, while others have shown acceleration of cognitive decline.

It appears that statins do not have a straight-line dose/toxicity relationship. Low doses appear to be more toxic (more likely to result in dementia) than high doses.

How do you spin such an uncomfortable finding? In this study, the way they camouflaged the results was to report that two of the drugs at high doses protected against dementia. What would have been more honest was to say that these two statins at high doses are not as brain toxic as the low dose statins. This would have to be supplemented with an explanation of a non-monotonic response, in a way that the ordinary non-medical person could grasp.

It is common practice to spin medical studies for the public media in such a way as to reflect favorably on a drug to boost sales. It is the specialty of drug company sales reps to "interpret" medical studies for doctors, and it certainly saves them the trouble of reading the articles themselves. Making matters worse are the many other ways that medical information gets funded by pharma, such as funding formal medical education, having a controlling interest in what research gets reported, and stacking advisory boards and committees that set national standards.

Your doctor is supposed to (by law) provide the opportunity for full informed consent, which would mean explaining all of this to you. But this almost never happens. So the responsibility lies with you, the patient, to get informed.

The bottom line is that the cumulative long-term effects of statin drugs on mental health *have not been adequately studied*. Certainly there is strong evidence that high cholesterol should be left alone in people age 70 and over.

CHAPTER 9

STATINS AND CANCER

It has long been observed that low cholesterol is associated with cancer. A 1992 article reviewed all earlier studies on the subject and reported that males with low cholesterol had a 30% increased risk of cancer; the most common types were colon, lung, and leukemia. Females with low cholesterol had a 5-10% increased risk of cancer; the most common types were breast, cervix, and leukemia. In contrast, other studies have suggested the risk of cancer in women on statins is greater than the risk for men on statins.

These correlations with cancer were based on studies of people who mostly had low cholesterol naturally, although some of them were on cholesterol-lowering drugs. The same researchers did a separate analysis of cancer risk in people who had low cholesterol only because they were treated with medications: the statistics on this focus group showed an increase in cancer occurrence of approximately 24%. [1] What can be concluded is that cholesterol low naturally or lowered by medication confers an increased chance of getting cancer.

Twenty years later, researchers discovered cancer cells have the capability of interfering with the normal movement of cholesterol across a cell membrane. It has not yet been sorted out what came first: cancer cells with their defective methods of handling cholesterol or abnormal levels of cholesterol promoting the growth of cancer cells. [2]

Since those early studies, there have been many more that looked at cancer risk from lowering cholesterol. British researchers looked at diseases in statin users and compared them to diseases in patients not on statins. They reported statins gave protection from getting esophageal cancer, *something not found by any other study before or since*. In fact, it is more likely that people on a statin drug are attempting to reduce their cardiac risk factors by not smoking—smoking is a major risk factor for the development of esophageal cancer. Just because the dog is in the hot-wired car, does not mean the dog stole the car.

Unlike other studies, the British researchers did not find an increased risk of any cancers; then again, they included patients as young as 30 years of age when cancers would be rare. [3] This is an example of how to design a study to get negative answers. Since most cancers are thought to take years to develop, it stands to reason that if you were looking for cancers, you would look in an older population. If you were looking for a drug effect, then you would look at people who had been on the drug for a long time. These days, some people remain on statins for decades. Instead, the British study included people as young as 30. Nonetheless, this faulty study is singled out in an attempt to negate the mounting evidence for statin-associated increased cancer risk.

The strength of the association of statin use to cancers heavily depends on age and duration of use, and to a small degree on gender and genetic background. The elderly are at highest risk from statin-associated cancers.

Remember, the PROSPER study done in 2002 was designed to look at the use of pravastatin in the elderly. It reported new cancers were 25% more likely in the elderly pravastatin-treated group than the elderly who were given a placebo. This demonstrates a statistically significant increase of cancer in those on the drug. In fact, any years of life gained by preventing a cardiovascular death were effectively cancelled out by the deaths from increased cancers. [4]

Two previous studies of pravastatin also showed increased new cancers. The PROPSER study authors tried to belittle the significance of the excess cancers by combining their statistics in a "meta-analysis" of past statin studies. By combining statistics of studies including subjects as young as 31 years of age, the cancer association in older subjects was obscured. Mixing in patients of much younger ages diluted any cancer trends that may have been present in the middle aged and elderly. The authors asserted that the excess cancers in their original study must have been "mere chance."

Yet another odd conclusion that should raise a suspicion of conflict of interest.

Major funding for the PROSPER study was provided by Bristol-Myers Squibb, who markets pravastatin, and 17 of the study's 20 authors had consultancy agreements and/or had received research support, fees, and/ or travel grants from various statin manufacturers or distributors.

Similarly, Bristol Myers Squibb funded the LIPID study of pravastatin. It followed subjects age 31 to 75 over the course of six years. The LIPID study authors reported no increase in the incidence of cancer. However, a separate sub-group analysis of only the elderly people in this study showed a significantly higher incidence in new cancers among elderly subjects on the drug. [5]

In 2007, another group—this time with no pharma funding—analyzed the combined data from 12 studies of pravastatin that reported on cancer incidence. They concluded pravastatin therapy was associated with an increasing risk of cancer as age increased. The mean age that started to show increased risk was 60. They called their conclusion "remarkably robust," meaning that their findings held up to intense scrutiny. [6] The take-away: the statistical analysis showing increased cancer is more reliable than any one of the pharma funded studies that attempted to refute it.

Pravastatin is not the only statin associated with increased new cancer incidence. Lipitor (atorvastatin) was the best selling statin drug in the world for many years. In a research project called Treating to New Targets (TNT study), high dose atorvastatin was compared to low dose statin. There was not a group on placebo. The study showed elderly subjects on high dose (80mg) atorvastatin had a trend toward increased deaths compared to those on a low dose (10mg) of the drug, and most of the deaths were from an increase in cancer. Although those on the higher dose atorvastatin had fewer cardiovascular deaths, they had increased deaths from other causes, including cancer. [7]

After more than two decades of experience with statin medications, a 2007 report described an analysis of the combined results from multiple studies of various patients on statin drugs. They selected cancer statistics from 23 different studies with publication dates ranging from 1991 though 2006. The report showed a strong relationship: the lower the LDL level achieved by the statins, the higher the incidence of new cancer diagnoses. [8]

Hold on, because it gets strange at this point.

The very next year, the same lead researchers issued a second report in which they claimed there was *no* relationship of statin treatment with new cancer diagnoses. In this paper, the authors did a re-analysis of many of the same studies used in the first paper, but dropped some of the original studies and added a few that had not been part of the first paper. In other words, it was a different mix of studies, and it makes a person wonder if they weren't cherry-picking the articles to review. Yet, the introduction and abstract summarizing of the research—which is all most doctors ever read and all most media ever report—give the distinct impression this new paper was a simple reanalysis of the very same group of studies reported on in the earlier article. [9]

The drastically different results in the second paper were generated not only by a remix of studies chosen for the analysis, but also by applying multiple layers of statistical manipulation based on so-called "meta-regression analysis." Meta-regression analysis techniques have gained popularity in the soft subjects of economics, behavioral experiments, and social studies. Since these fields involve human behavior, they don't lend themselves to strictly scientific analysis. Meta-regression analysis is a series of mathematical equations supposed to remove the effects of variation among studies of differing designs. It is intended to homogenize the results, and like homogenized food, all of the disagreeable elements are blended in until they are no longer detectable. That is exactly what happened: anything obvious about statins linked to cancer just dropped out.

Drug studies do not belong in the soft sciences category because outcomes in drug studies are distinctly measurable and not about human *behaviors* that method is designed to stabilize. The unusual application of meta-regression analytics to dilute negative results leads to suspicion of conflict of interest. One of the lead authors of the first paper was Dr. Richard Karas, listed in that paper as having potential conflicts of interest. He received research grants from AstraZeneca and Kos Pharmaceuticals; served on the speakers' bureaus of and/or received fees from Kos, AstraZeneca, Merck, and Pfizer; and served as a consultant to Kos Pharmaceuticals. In the later paper, Dr. Karas was again listed as being a recipient of funds from statin-manufacturers. However, unlike the first article, co-author Dr. Alsheikh-Ali was newly listed as being the recipient of funds from a statin manufacturer. Another lead researcher, Dr. Kent, also had financial ties to three statin makers. The later (2008) article includes these disclosures: "Dr. Alsheikh-Ali is currently a recipient of a faculty development award from Pfizer/Tufts Medical Center. Dr. Kent has received research support from Pfizer. Dr. Karas has received honoraria from Merck and Abbott, and research support from AstraZeneca."

In the second paper, the authors do not directly say their earlier findings of the cancer-statin link were wrong. However, they had to make some attempt at explaining away the vastly differing results of their 2008 analysis, so they stated: "The interpretation of these findings and their implications for understanding the observed inverse association between on-treatment LDL-C levels and incident cancer remain complex..."

Ah yes, it is all very complex. A better explanation might be that you can make anything seem to disappear by manipulating what information becomes part of the statistics.

There are a few large studies on statins, cholesterol, and specific types of cancer, and they can be conflicting. For example, two 2013 publications in the same journal gave vastly different conclusions about statin use and the risk of breast cancer. The first paper looked at women age 55 to 74 living in the Seattle area; patients with invasive breast cancer were compared with women who did not have cancer. Women who were currently using statins and had been for 10 years or longer had an 83% higher risk of getting invasive ductal cancer and nearly double the risk of invasive lobular cancer compared with women who never used statins. The Seattle researchers took a further step and analyzed the cancer risk in just the women who were diagnosed with high cholesterol per NCEP guidelines. They found that if these women with initially high cholesterol were statin users of more than 10 years, they had an even higher risk of breast cancer than the group of statin users as a whole. Women with a diagnosis of high cholesterol who were on statins had double the risk of invasive ductal carcinoma, and 2.4-fold higher risk of invasive lobular carcinoma compared to patients who never used statins. [10] Stated another way, people who had high cholesterol to begin with, and took statin drugs for that high cholesterol, had even greater risk of breast cancer than statin users who didn't have a diagnosis of high cholesterol. This result has provoked a line of research to see if high cholesterol is specifically protective against breast cancer.

Just a few months later, the very same journal published the findings of the Women's Health Initiative (WHI) study with vastly different conclusions. The WHI study followed women ages 50 to 79 for an average of nearly 11 years. It reported that the annualized, or average yearly rate of breast cancer, was no greater in statin users. How could this study give such different results than the Seattle study described above?

One of the major differences was the duration of statin use. In the Seattle study showing significantly increased cancer risk, statin use was ten years or more and current. In the Women's Health Initiative study, one-third were on statins for less than one year, one-third were on statins for 1-3 years, and only one-third were on statins for more than three years. In fact, the Seattle study provides a much more accurate measure of breast cancer risk for long term current statin users than the Women's Health Initiative study. [11]

The vastly differing results of these studies demonstrate that research projects can be carefully designed to minimize potentially embarrassing results for statin manufacturers. The first article, showing a clearly increased cancer risk in long-term current statin users, was sponsored by a grant from the National Cancer Institute and its authors had no conflicts of interest. Authors of the *second* article, which showed no cancer relationship, included one Lisa Martin, who received commercial research grants from four statin manufacturers (Amarin, Amgen, Sanofi, and Novartis). Of course, the second article was not *designed* to measure the effect of long-term statin use. The WHI study only followed patients for a very short time, so the study cannot possibly answer the question about long-term cancer risk in statin users.

A British newspaper headline in 2014 read that lowering cholesterol might *prevent* breast cancer. This was based on the preliminary results of an as yet unpublished study that found women with high cholesterol had 64% increased risk of breast cancer. First of all, there is no indication that the researchers even looked at whether treatment with statins reduced breast cancer risk. Second, and most important, there is no information about statin use by these women with high cholesterol. If the Seattle study results are applicable, then it is likely the English study will also show the typical chain of events: women with high cholesterol get treated with statins, and those on statins for high cholesterol have an increased risk of cancer. Attributing increased risk of breast cancer to the fact of high cholesterol alone is a simplistic view that ignores decades of proof of the relationship of low cholesterol to cancers, including breast cancer, and the more recent studies showing nearly double the risk of breast cancer with long term statin use. [12]

There have been inconsistent reports about the effect of statins on the incidence of colon cancer, with some studies showing a protective effect and others showing no effect. [13]

In one report, researchers combined the statistics from many studies to look at the combined rates of cancer of the colon, breast, and lung. They compared statin users to comparable patients not on statins. No increased cancers or decreased cancers were found in the statin group. However, two great weaknesses of the study make these results very questionable:

the statin users were younger than the average age in the control group, and the mean follow up was less than three years. [14] This is another good example of how to design a study to get a null answer. If you do not want to find increased cancers, then look at younger people who have a shorter duration of statin use, and then only follow them for 3 years or less.

> *According to Mark Twain, "There are three kinds of lies: lies, damned lies, and statistics."* [15]

The studies of prostate cancer and statins are likewise not clear-cut. In 2012, a combined analysis was done on the statistics from 27 studies reporting on statin use and prostate cancer. The studies included men from relatively young to elderly, with various other illnesses, on a variety of different statin medications and doses, and for varying lengths of time. Some studies showed increased prostate cancer risk, others showed decreased risk, and some showed no effect on risk of prostate cancer. In the study that showed the greatest protective effect (nearly 80% reduction in the incidence of new prostate cancers), the duration of statin use was the shortest at about 3 years. In the study that showed the greatest harmful effect (40% *increased* risk of prostate cancer in statin users) the duration of statin use was over ten years.

The cumulative results showed a 7% protective effect of statin use on initial prostate cancer, but statistically was majorly due to the single study showing a nearly 80% decreased prostate cancer incidence. In other words, that one study was so unlike the other studies that it gave undue weight to the combined analysis. The authors admitted long-term statin use was *not* protective against prostate cancer. [16]

The very next year, another study failed to confirm any protective effect of statins on the risk of prostate cancer recurrence after initial surgery. 1,200 men with prostate cancer treated with prostate removal were followed for 5 years. The statin use of the ones who developed recurrent prostate cancer was compared to statin use in the ones who remained free of cancer. No protective effect of statins could be identified. [17]

In summary, statins appear to cause an increased risk for breast cancer in women, cancer in general in the elderly, and cancers in people taking high doses or in *anyone* taking statins over a long period of time.

CHAPTER 10

STATINS AND DIABETES

Statin drugs lead to an increase in diabetes. Diabetes, in turn, is a strong risk factor for the development of all forms of cardiovascular disease, including heart attack and stroke. Diabetics also have reduced lifespans from all causes. If that seems unbelievable to you, let's put it another way:

Statin drugs, which may be a minor risk factor for a heart attack, can cause diabetes, which shortens lifespan overall and is a major risk factor for heart attack.

It has been known for at least 25 years that statin drugs promote new onset of diabetes. Statins impair the function of specialized cells in the pancreas that secrete insulin, the hormone that controls the body's use of sugars. While a person is on statins, the circulating insulin levels actually increase, but the cells are less responsive to the insulin. Thus, glucose, which insulin should pull into the cells, remains in the circulation resulting in diabetes. Women, Asians, and the elderly are especially prone to develop diabetes while on statins. [1]

So here we have a drug promoting the development of diabetes, yet diabetes itself (independent of cholesterol levels) is associated with premature death. The US Cancer Prevention Study enrolled over one million adults and followed them for a 26-year period. Compared to people who were not diabetic, diabetes was found to be associated with higher risks of death involving the circulatory system, respiratory system, digestive system, genitourinary system, and external causes/accidental deaths, as well as having a higher risk of death from cancer. Among women, diabetes was found to be associated with higher risk of death from cancers of the liver, pancreas, uterus, colon, and breast. Among men, diabetes was associated with risk of death from cancers of the breast, liver, mouth and throat, pancreas, bladder, and colon. [2]

Given the increased cancer risk for diabetics even before they are put on statin drugs, the added effects of statins has to be examined even more closely. In addition to driving excess insulin (hormone that regulates sugar) secretion and impairing insulin sensitivity, statin therapy causes increased levels of another hormone called *inulin* (a storage form of sugar), and increased production of *insulin-like growth factor*. When these two substances are present in normal amounts, they contribute to the balanced regulation of cell division and growth. When there is too much of them, cell division can go awry. This chain of events is thought to contribute to plaque growth on the linings of arteries, which leads to heart attacks, as well as to the growth of cancers. [3]

Anyone who has already had a heart attack is more likely to suffer another one. But diabetics who haven't yet had a heart attack are just as likely to have one as non-diabetics who have already had a heart attack. Patients with diabetes have chronic low-grade inflammation of their arterial lining, probably related to excess sugar in the bloodstream and elevated levels of insulin.

Since people who are already diabetic have an increased risk for heart disease; it seems reasonable to recommend they be on statins, at least at first—until you add up the drug side effects. But remember, statins are being widely prescribed to prevent heart attacks in people who aren't diabetic. However, the drug itself may create diabetes, so it makes this rationale look awfully backwards.

In 2012, researchers reported on the incidence of diabetes in postmenopausal women on statin drugs. The Women's Health Initiative was a twenty-year (and ongoing) study following the health of 153,840 women who were not diabetic at the start. Women on statins had a significantly increased risk of developing diabetes—they were 70% more likely to become diabetic than women not on statins. [4]

So with all of the information saying not to, why would statins be prescribed to people at risk for or with diabetes? It is because some studies conclude diabetics on statins live longer despite the adverse drug effects, but other studies do not substantiate this finding. It is argued that the small reduction in cardiovascular deaths overcomes the negative effects of those developing diabetes because of the drug. A useful way to sort out conflicting study conclusions is to combine the results of the studies and see what the overall numbers tell us. When the combined results of 14 different studies of diabetics on statins were analyzed, there was a reduction of death overall compared to diabetics not on statins; this was almost entirely due to reductions in death from cardiovascular disease. From this we can definitely say that in the short term, statins are good for people who are already diabetic. The weakness of this analysis is that the follow up was only a mean of 4.3 years. In other words, it does not mirror the real life situation where people are put on statins for decades. What we are most concerned about with diabetes is the *long-term* adverse effects, such as blindness, kidney failure, leg amputations, painful neuropathy, and premature death. A follow up period of 4.3 years could never detect these things. As with so many other studies, this analysis was not designed to measure the risk in real life situations when people are on statins very long-term. [5]

When non-diabetics use statins, the treatment does not slow the rate of plaque build up in the arteries. Since diabetics already tend to get hardening of the arteries at an accelerated rate, researchers were especially interested to see if statins slowed the process in them. 197 veterans with diabetes who already had advanced calcification of their major vessels were studied. Measurements were taken to determine the degree of calcification in their coronary arteries and in the aorta (the main vessel that comes from the heart and delivers blood to the body). Their medical records were reviewed to see how much of the time they were taking their statins as prescribed. The diabetics who took their statin medication more closely as prescribed had lower cholesterol levels and near perfect LDL levels. However, the progression of coronary artery calcification and abdominal aortic artery calcification was *accelerated* according to the frequency of statin use—the more frequent the use of statins, the *faster* the arteries calcified. [6]

Elevated blood sugar is only one aspect of diabetes. Diabetics can experience vision abnormalities even before the blood sugar becomes abnormal, and remain at higher risk for all of the main causes of blindness (macular degeneration, cataracts, and glaucoma). In a study of 452 patients with type-2 diabetes, it was found that diabetics on statin drugs had a significantly increased incidence of cataracts compared to diabetics not on statins. [7]

Diabetics commonly suffer from a disorder of the nerves in the hands and feet called *peripheral neuropathy*. This can be painful, lead to complete loss of normal feeling, and be complicated by deformities in the foot bones and ulcers on the legs and feet. There are insufficient studies on the role of statins in promoting neuropathy in diabetics. However, regardless of diabetes, population studies have clearly demonstrated statin use is associated with neuropathy in general. Despite the FDA-mandated warning on the package inserts of all statin drugs, the diagnosis of statin-associated neuropathy is likely under-recognized in diabetics. Pain and numbness in a diabetic is much more likely to be attributed to diabetic neuropathy with no further consideration that it could be due to the statin drug they are taking. This is especially true since statin-induced neuropathy may not occur until after being on the drug for two years or more, further facilitating a direct association easily being missed.

Diabetes commonly leads to kidney disease and even kidney failure and is the number one underlying disease in people on dialysis. People who take high doses of statins (or an especially potent statin) are more likely to develop serious kidney problems than people on a more usual dose. If statins were prescribed for diabetics, high doses would be expected to make them at particular risk for kidney disease on top of their risk from the diabetes alone.

In summary, statins promote several major complications of diabetes, as well as promoting the development of new diabetes and the worsening of blood sugar control in existing diabetics.

CHAPTER 11

OTHER NOTORIOUS STATIN SIDE EFFECTS

There are yet additional serious adverse effects of statin drugs. Investigators in England looked into the patient files of over 225,000 statin users. They found definite increased risk of moderate or serious liver dysfunction, acute kidney failure, moderate or serious muscle damage, and cataracts compared to people not on statins. [1] Statin nerve damage is another common unwanted drug effect. Let's take a closer look at each of these.

Statin Myopathy

Myopathy is a general term meaning any abnormality of the muscles. Statin-associated myopathy is not well understood though it is considered one of the most severe adverse effects of these drugs. The patient can develop muscle aches and pains and lab work shows elevated levels of muscle protein enzymes, reflecting muscle damage and breakdown. Mild myopathy may not show elevated enzymes on blood tests, but nevertheless, the patient feels sore and fatigued.

When muscle breakdown is massive it is called *rhabdomyolysis*, a medical word of Greek origin that literally means the destruction of muscle fibers. Urine turns brown and especially stinky and there are continuous painful muscle cramps, weakness, and profound fatigue. In severe cases, muscle proteins can be circulating in such high levels that they actually clog the kidneys and result in permanent kidney failure or death. The usual treatment is to stop the statins while supporting the kidneys with intravenous fluids, but some advanced myopathies are not reversible even when the statin is discontinued. [2]

In a study on rats given atorvastatin, damage to the muscles was found to include disorganized and misshapen muscle cells, clumps of dead muscle tissue, shrunken cell nuclei, dismantled cell membranes, and fatty deposits in muscles. [3]

Medical literature routinely puts the incidence of statin-associated myopathy at only 1% to 5%, but most doctors in clinical practice will report seeing it much more frequently. Some studies give numbers showing a quarter to more than a third of patients who take statins will sooner or later develop a clinically significant myopathy. Women and the elderly are more often affected. [4]

Myopathy is also more likely to occur on high dose statins, in patients over 60, in those who have underlying kidney or liver disease, in alcoholics, or in anyone who is dehydrated. Low thyroid and vitamin D deficiency can also promote this side effect. There is an extensive list of medications that make myopathy more likely if the person is also on statins, including other cholesterol lowering drugs, medications to inhibit stomach acid, and some blood thinners.

Myopathy can occur while on any statin, at any dose. In general, the higher the statin dose, the greater the risk of myopathy. The dose relationship is not a hard and fast rule because some very potent statins that also last longest in the body may cause myopathy at a dose lower than less potent drugs. The other factor is that the more easily the statin passes into muscle, the more likely it is to cause myopathy. The risk of statin myopathy is least with pravastatin, increasingly more risky for fluvastatin, then rosuvastatin and atorvastatin, and is most likely with lovastatin or simvastatin.

The interplay of genetics is getting a lot of attention for playing a role in the risk of myopathy. Specifically, the lack of certain genes makes statin-induced myopathy more likely. Genetic tendency is increasingly being blamed, but of all the genetic types chased down, only two have been definitely related to an increased risk for myopathy. The vast majority of people who get muscle inflammation from statins do not have either of these rare genetic defects. Genetic testing is available to determine in advance who would be at highest risk for statin myopathy, but it is almost never done. [5]

Cholesterol is an important structural element to the membranes and walls of cells, and has a functional role in controlling the flow of ordinary biochemicals back and forth through the cell wall. Statins reduce the cholesterol content of skeletal muscle cell membranes and this might make them leaky, unstable, and tend to collapse. Other theories about how statins cause myopathy relate to abnormally massive shifts of calcium across cell membranes and the production of antibodies that cross-react with muscle tissue, attacking it. [6]

Regardless of genetics, statins are known to deplete the level of circulating coQ10. Low coQ10, in turn, can make muscle pain more likely. The proof of this is seen when someone with statin-induced myopathy is given extra coQ10: supplementing with coQ10 (50 mg twice a day) can relieve symptoms of myopathy in many people. [7]

Many patients are not officially diagnosed with statin-associated myopathy because although they complain of muscle pains, their muscle enzymes are not elevated as high as 10-fold, which is required for the diagnosis. They are either diagnosed with *myositis* (muscle inflammation) or ignored altogether. There is not adequate information on the long-term consequences of low-level myositis from statins. Sadly, undiagnosed statin myositis can progress all the way to making the patient wheelchair-bound while they continue taking their daily dose of statin. One group of researchers warned that if progressive muscle symptoms are ignored, deaths can occur. [8]

A large study of veterans demonstrated that exercise lowered the risk of death from cardiovascular disease at least as much as statins did. It is ironic then that statin therapy is associated with a high incidence of fatigue and intolerance to exercise. Is it justified to give a pill that will prevent participation in an entirely safe, non-drug means of life extension? [9]

Statin Associated Liver Injury

Any statin can cause a rise of the circulating levels of liver enzymes. These are substances usually present in the circulation in low amounts, and tend to rise only when there is liver cell irritation or injury. On blood test results, these are called *alanine aminotransferase* (ALT) and *aspartate aminotransferase* (AST). Some studies showed that in about 70% of patients, the enzyme levels return to normal even while continuing the statin. However, when the enzymes stay elevated, it is necessary to lower the dose of statin or stop the statin altogether; they will usually return to normal levels, but not in all people. Unfortunately, enzyme elevation can only be detected through routine liver tests, which is not required by the FDA.

In April 2006, the National Lipid Association's Statin Safety Task Force reported on statin toxicity. The four-member safety task force was funded by grants from manufacturers or distributors of statins, including Abbott, AstraZeneca, Kos Pharmaceuticals, and Merck/Schering-Plough. In addition, the three liver experts consulted by the task force had been in the pay of statin manufacturers.

In their section on liver toxicity, the task force reported the incidence of liver failure was no greater among statin users than in people not on statins. In the studies they reviewed to draw their conclusions, many patients were not counted because they had immediate elevation of liver enzymes within the first few weeks; those patients were excluded from all further statistical analysis. It is convenient when a drug causes adverse effects in the first few weeks to call this time frame the "run-in period" and omit counting drug effects in final results. [10] This does not give enough information for real life scenarios where liver-sensitive patients tend to be continued on statin drugs despite increased liver enzymes, positioning the doctor to make a decision that subjects his patient to potentially severe liver damage.

When asked if enzyme elevations indicate liver damage, the liver experts answered "no." But when asked if taking statins increases the chance of liver failure, liver transplants, or death, they gave a qualified "yes," explaining this was a "rare" side effect. In January 2014, the FDA changed its recommendations and stopped advising routine liver enzyme testing for statin users. [11] It seems to be a situation of "Don't ask. Don't tell." If the liver tests are never measured, then liver abnormalities from statin drugs will never be detected or reported.

The direct relationship of statins to liver irritation is illustrated by studies showing the higher the dose of statins, the greater the chance of liver enzyme elevation. In one study of atorvastatin, those on a high dose had three times the risk of liver enzyme elevation compared to those on a low dose. [12] Meanwhile, researchers continue to document the liver-damaging effects of statin drugs. When simvastatin was added to liver cell cultures in the laboratory setting, it caused liver cell inflammation, cell death, increased damage from byproducts of normal metabolism, decreased manufacture of cellular energy, and decreased levels of coQ10. [13] When liver cells were incubated with any of the most commonly used statins (atorvastatin, lovastatin, or simvastatin) researchers found several indicators of cell damage and increased cell death. The higher the statin concentration, the greater the cellular damage. [14]

Physician awareness of common and serious statin side effects is very low, even when their patients distinctly describe their symptoms. [15] One survey of 650 patients on statin drugs found that when patients complained to their doctors about muscle weakness or pain, or mentioned cognitive problems such as memory loss and other symptoms, physicians dismissed the possibility of adverse drug reactions nearly a third of the time. Even when elevations of liver enzymes were found, they were not often attributed to statin use. In addition to doctors saying, "That's not a side effect of this drug," the complaining patients got these responses:

"You can expect some problems at your age."

"Doctor suggested it was my imagination."

"Doctor said I would have to live with the side effects and did not seem to care."

"Doctor said…only 1% of patients have side effects." [16]

Statins and Cataracts

Researchers looked into databases of electronic medical information in the US, UK, and Canada to compare the relationships of statin use to the need for cataract surgery. The increased risk for cataracts in statin users in the US database was 7%; that is statistically significant, leading to the conclusion that statins are definitely a risk for the development of cataracts. Nearly four times that risk was found among people in the Canadian database: those who took statins for at least a year had nearly 27% increased risk of developing cataracts needing surgery compared with people not taking statins. [17]

In the most conservative cataract study, thousands of people who had cataract surgery were compared to those not needing cataract surgery, and their statin use was recorded. The results depended on age:

- over age 65, a greater proportion of those on statin drugs needed cataract surgery; this is precisely the age group that is at highest risk of dying from a heart attack and therefore most likely to be prescribed statins

- age 50-63, the use of statins was associated with fewer cataract surgeries as long as they were on the drugs for at least 4 to 5 years

In other words, statins seemed to protect against cataracts in the younger age group, but promote catacts in the older group. The absolute best that can be said about statins and cataracts is: statin use is likely to harm the elderly. These mixed results are in line with many other studies showing a waning beneficial effect of statins as people get older. [18]

In a study regarding glaucoma, people on statins were found to have a slightly decreased chance of getting glaucoma, but the results were slight and not strongly in favor of any protective effect. [19] Although these results were not statistically significant, the headlines screamed that statins could prevent glaucoma. Meanwhile, the FDA's Adverse Drug Event Reporting System logged reports of individuals on statins suffering other eye abnormalities, including loss of movement of the eyeball, upper lid drooping, and double vision. In each case, the effect resolved when the statin was stopped. [20] Reporting of adverse drug events is a massive under-representation of what is really happening, with an estimated 75-85% of drug side effects never being reported at all. [21]

Statins and Kidney Injury

Statins have long been associated with kidney injury, but large manufacturer-sponsored studies have not shown a strong correlation with their drugs. In such studies, it is left up to the participating research doctor to assign a cause to any episodes of kidney injury. In a company-sponsored study, isn't a tendency to miss-assign cause information a possibility? Maybe even probablity? A way around these overt or subtle conflicts of interest is to use health databases to simply count the rate of a certain side effect in a large population on the drugs.

The study conducted in England and Wales mentioned earlier found a 50% increase in acute kidney failure among people on any statins within the first year of use. The risk for kidney failure was greater when dosage was higher. [22]

In another recent study, researchers looked through the health databases of over 2 million patients in Canada, the US, and the UK. They found that in people who didn't have any pre-existing kidney issues, those on high dose or high potency statins were 34% more likely to be hospitalized for acute kidney injury within 120 days after starting statin treatment. In this study, *high potency* was defined as 10 mg or more of rosuvastatin, 20 mg or more of atorvastatin, and 40 mg or more of simvastatin; all other statin treatments were defined as low potency. For patients who already had existing chronic kidney disease, there was also an increased risk of hospitalization because of further kidney injury. [23]

In summary, high dose statins and high potency statins are associated with a significantly increased risk of acute kidney injury so severe as to require hospitalization.

Statins and Neuropathy

The association between statins and neuropathy is also well established. A large US study showed the prevalence of peripheral neuropathy was significantly higher among those who used statins compared with those not on statins. When the US National Health and Nutrition Survey was examined, it was found that the incidence of peripheral neuropathy (affecting the nerves in the legs) was 23.5% in those who used statins, compared to only 13.5% in those who did not. The statin association remained strong even when the statistics were controlled for other conditions that could lead to neuropathy, such as diabetes, alcohol abuse, and vitamin deficiencies. [24]

In an even more remarkable study, Danish researchers found that people taking statins were 14 times more likely to develop peripheral neuropathy than people who were not taking statins, especially if they were on the drugs for more than two years. Incredibly, even with evidence like this, some doctors are so enthusiastic about statin use that they suggest this "14 times more likely" incidence of neuropathy may be due to chance! [25]

CHAPTER 12

NEW CHOLESTEROL DRUGS:
THE PCSK9 ANTIBODIES

The very newest drugs to be marketed for reducing cholesterol have a novel mechanism of action unrelated to the statins. Normally, special receptors get rid of excess LDL in the bloodstream as it passes through the liver. LDL latches onto liver LDL receptors that facilitate disposal. These receptors are only useful for a limited time. An elaborate feedback mechanism seems to signal the body to deactivate the LDL receptors. This is done by a biochemical with an impossible name, so it is commonly abbreviated as PCSK9 and pronounced *pic-sic-nine*.

The new anti-cholesterol drugs attack PCSK9, so nothing is there to decommission LDL receptors. This leaves the body with extra LDL receptors. It works: the extra LDL receptors result in clearing more LDL out of the bloodstream.

Alirocumab (Praluent) and evolocumab (Repatha) are antibodies with specific activity against PCSK9. The drugs are manufactured using a biochemical factory: live cultures of hamster ovary cells are programmed with DNA to generate massive reproduction of the antibodies. It is a type of cloning—the culture cells churn out billions of exact duplicates of these designer antibodies. Both drugs have *–mab* at the end of their chemical names to represent *monoclonal antibodies*, meaning a massive clone of a single kind of antibody, artificially produced in identical cells.

At first, the drugs were studied only in rare conditions caused by inherited genetic mutations resulting in extremely high cholesterol levels in afflicted family members. Then, studies extended to heart patients with LDL levels remaining above guidelines even on statin drugs. This is the group that made the expensive drug development worthwhile, especially since guidelines for "acceptable" LDL levels keep getting revised downward.

As is usual for a new class of drugs, the PCSK9 antibody drugs were approved by the FDA after only short term studies, with most only lasting 24 weeks and few over two years. These are injectable drugs self-administered by the patient once every two to four weeks at a cost of over $14,000 per year at the time of their approvals in 2015. Besides the side effect of draining the Medicare Trust Fund, the common adverse effects reported in the drug-makers' studies include injection site reaction and allergic reaction, as well as:

sore throat	muscle pain
cough	muscle spasm
upper respiratory tract infection	bruising
sinus infection	joint pain
flu	dizziness
headache	high blood pressure
fatigue	nause
back pain	diarrhea
urinary tract infection	gastroenteritis [1,2]

The manufacturer-sponsored studies do not report a significant incidence of mental effects, but the data does suggest there may be some tendency for brain impairment. The FDA is concerned enough that it has required manufacturers to continue following a subset of the experimental patients and to conduct neurological testing on them well into the future. [3]

Animal studies show that PCSK9 can promote brain cell death. This might suggest that an antibody drug against PCSK9 could possibly prevent Alzheimer's dementia. However, the same studies also show PCSK9 can act to inhibit brain cell death. In that case, knocking out PCSK9 could lead to more Alzheimer's. [4]

*The bottom line: we have a powerful new drug with little research
and no long term data that could be a double-edged sword.*

Rarely a study patient was reported to have extremely low LDL levels (less than 25 mg/dL). The Repatha package insert admits the consequences of such low LDL levels are "not known" though there are many studies showing an association between low cholesterol levels and increased incidence of cancer and dementia, as covered in an earlier chapter. [5]

The variation in how well the drug works and its side effects in the elderly and across various races are difficult to determine. This is because the study statistics tend to be reported on diverse groups. Studies included age ranges from 18 to 74 and involved relatively few non-Caucasians. There also may be some differences in how these drugs work between males and females. Animal studies show that when PCSK9 is low, it raises the number of LDL receptors in the liver in men more than in premenopausal women, who tend to have more LDL receptors show up in the gut and fat tissue. Both sexes have increases in LDL receptors in the pancreas. [6]

The long-term effects of changing the number of LDL receptors in various organs are not known. In the pancreas, for instance, increased LDL receptors cause an unusually high concentration of cholesterol to accumulate there. The pancreas makes insulin in response to high blood sugar, but high cholesterol levels in the pancreas have been associated with faulty release of enough insulin. [7]

Some patients have developed antibodies to the drugs. While the drugs themselves are antibodies, the human body can recognize them as foreign and make antibodies against the drugs. The long-term consequences of these anti-antibodies are not known. It is also unknown whether it is safe to continue taking the drugs once those anti-antibodies have been detected. Other types of monoclonal antibody drugs used in cancer treatment, viral hepatitis, and autoimmune conditions have shown complications such as heart damage, provoking system-wide immune reactions, and increasing the risk of getting cancer. [8]

Yes, you did just read that right. These drugs have the potential to cause exactly what they claim to treat.

In summary, information from the limited duration human studies and more extensive animal testing suggests the PCSK9 antibody drugs may *eventually* be found to increase diabetes, cause the development of autoimmune disease in some people, and result in brain malfunction in sensitive persons over the long term.

It is important to remember that just because high LDL has been associated with an increased risk of heart disease in some populations, it is not a major risk factor as described in depth in an earlier chapter. In fact, in some families with a genetic mutation that causes extremely high LDL levels, there is no increase in heart disease compared to the rest of the population. [9] So to apply a "one-size fits most" recommendation for drug treatments in a broader patient population is not warranted.

Although the PCSK9 antibody drugs are effective at lowering LDL, so far there is no evidence that they reduce heart attacks or strokes, and they have not been proven to prolong life. And here's an interesting fact:

Regular exercise has been shown to naturally reduce PCSK9 activity and result in lower LDL levels with virtually no side effects! [10]

CHAPTER 13

ALTERNATIVES FOR LOWERING
CARDIOVASCULAR DISEASE RISK

This chapter is not about using alternatives to lower cholesterol. As you have learned, cholesterol is probably only a minor risk factor in some people, and not a risk factor at all for many.

Hardening of the arteries, or atherosclerosis, is characterized by plaque build-up in the vessels. Plaque is made up of fibrous tissue, fat, cholesterol, calcium crystals, and collagen. Within plaque is a center of dead tissue, and throughout the plaque are various kinds of inflammatory cells. Bacteria are also present in a large proportion of plaques. Several different lines of investigation have converged on the conclusion that plaque build-up in arteries is but a residual of a chronic inflammatory process. To blame cholesterol, which is just one of the many components of plaque, is like blaming calcium for arthritis: we do find calcium deposits in the joints of arthritis sufferers, but calcium is the body's *response* to inflammation, not the *cause* of it. Removing cholesterol makes about as much sense as performing a hysterectomy (surgical removal of the womb) for the treatment of hysteria, a practice that existed well into the 19th century.

The emphasis on the study and treatment of hardening of the arteries (atherosclerosis) has been on the physical blockage. It would be much better to work on the real causes leading to blockage. There is a lot of scientific support for atherosclerosis being an inflammatory condition. The blood of people with arterial plaques contains high levels of various inflammatory markers. These include substances called C-reactive protein (CRP), amyloid A, and interleukins. Alternative treatments have focused on following these markers to address existing inflammation and reduce the development of inflammatory deposits.

This is not meant as a comprehensive list of all heart protective possibilities. It is just enough to let you know that you can do many things to protect your heart and maintain health despite the genes you've been dealt, your cholesterol level, and your doctor's insistence on statin drugs. Information on alternatives to suggested treatments is a component of full informed consent.

Reducing Major Risk Factors

Cholesterol appears to be a minor risk factor for heart disease and only so in some people. In contrast, there are some major risk factors that can be controlled.

1. Don't smoke. Smoking lowers the good heart-protective HDL cholesterol, damages heart muscle, and raises blood pressure.

2. High blood pressure that goes untreated causes undue strain on the heart muscle and damages arteries. High blood pressure should be treated.

3. Insulin resistance and its consequences (such as diabetes) are preventable and reversible conditions in the majority of people. Most disorders of insulin metabolism can be reversed with weight reduction, exercise, and a low-carbohydrate way of eating.

4. Obesity is a major risk that may have many different contributing factors including genetics, stress, and low activity level, but it *always* responds to a restricted calorie diet.

Exercise

Regular physical activity stresses the heart in a good way by stimulating a healthy cardiovascular system. Exercise benefits the blood flow, conditions the heart pumping action, and supports normalization of blood pressure even before it produces any weight loss or muscle strengthening. Some studies have suggested the exercise rehab program after heart bypass surgery is more responsible for good outcomes than the operation itself. [1]

Diets

The body makes almost all of the cholesterol it has in circulation. The idea that the fats we eat cause high cholesterol levels, or that a low-fat diet will lower heart disease risk, is only weakly supported by scientific evidence. Let's take a closer look at diets with various theories of optimum fat intake.

In 1958, nutrition researcher Ancel Keys found that men from the Greek island of Crete and from villages in Southern Italy had a lower incidence of heart disease than men in several other countries. There could have been many factors involved, including the active lifestyle of fishermen and farmers in those regions, but being a nutrition researcher, Keys decided it was diet related. His reports popularized the so-called Mediterranean diet, which includes a high intake of olive oil, fruit, nuts, vegetables, and grains; a moderate intake of fish and poultry; a low intake of dairy products, sweets, red meat, and processed meats; and wine in moderation, consumed with meals. [2]

A study in 2013 compared subjects on a Mediterranean diet consuming fat from olive oils or nuts to subjects on a modified American low-fat diet. There was a lower incidence of cardiovascular events (heart attack, stroke, or death from cardiovascular event) by 1%: a one percentage point advantage for the people eating the Mediterranean diet. But, the study was flawed because it turned out that the American 'low-fat' diet group was not really adhering to low-fat, such that the compared groups actually ate a similar amount of fat and red meats. [3] The bottom line is that food rules do not seem to be separable from lifestyle factors when evaluating the effect on overall heart health. However, it is noteworthy that Dr. Keys, born in 1904, followed the Mediterranean diet and lived to see his hundredth birthday before passing in 2004.

Sixty years after the work of Keys, we have the capacity to track and analyze much larger international data sets. In 2008, when Dr. Malcolm Kendrick studied the World Health Organization's statistics on death rates from various causes, he got results that upset the prevailing low-fat diet fads. Kendrick found that the seven countries with the *lowest* consumption of saturated fats had *higher* rates of heart disease than the countries with the highest consumption of saturated fats. This information completely undermines the low-fat diet recommendations of organizations such as the American Heart Association. [4]

Dr. Dean Ornish made news headlines in 1990 when a study was published demonstrating major lifestyle changes, including the Ornish diet, not only halted but reversed plaque buildup in arteries. The Ornish diet is low in fat from foods (comprising only 10% of daily calories), but includes taking fatty fish oil supplements. Meat is avoided (both red and white), as is sugar in any refined form. The Ornish plan is high in fiber and includes plenty of fish and unlimited fruits, beans, and vegetables. The Ornish plan also includes major lifestyle modifications consisting of exercise, stress reduction, and avoiding negativity. A follow-up study showed a high rate of continuing adherence to the Ornish plan and demonstrated that not only was the initial weight loss maintained, but the regression of vessel blockage also continued. It has not been determined if the low-fat component of the diet is incidental to the results, or if the low sugar consumption is really the major dietary factor in decreasing vessel inflammation. For all we know, it could be lifestyle modifications having the largest effect, but there is no doubt that hardening of the arteries regresses on the Ornish plan. [5]

In the 1970s, cardiologist Dr. Robert Atkins was severely attacked by the American Medical Association for his claims that it was not fat causing weight gain and heart disease, but carbohydrates like breads, pasta, refined products, and sugar. The Atkins diet turns the government's food pyramid on its head: Atkins diet is high in protein with limited carbohydrates, but no restrictions on fat. Science has borne out Dr. Atkins' assertions. There are hundreds of scientific studies that identify a cascade of inflammatory events are triggered by consumption of unrefined carbs, and particularly sugar. Restricted carbohydrate diets that do not limit fat actually improve metabolic syndrome and diabetes even before any weight is lost. [6] The high-fat/low-carb diet was criticized when Dr. Atkins suffered cardiomyopathy in the year 2000. This condition is characterized by heart muscle weakness, not hardening of the arteries. In fact, Atkins' arteries were checked at that time and found to be clean. When Atkins died in 2003, it was from a head injury after slipping on the ice following a snow storm.

Today's popular Paleo diets are another modification on low-carb diets. The general Paleo diet allows lean meats, fish, eggs, fruits, vegetables, nuts, seeds, and healthier oils (such as coconut oil and olive oil). Paleo dieters avoid grains and any processed foods such as breads. Dairy, peanuts, beans, refined sugar, potatoes, and salt are also avoided. It is a low-inflammation kind of diet, but objective studies regarding the effect of a Paleo diet on heart health have not yet been done.

Sugars and refined carbohydrates readily converted to simple sugars cause the body to pump more insulin into circulation. It is the job of insulin to get the sugar into the cells where it is stored as fat. Undesirable aspects of insulin can be seen when the circulating levels are very high. Insulin's damaging effects include excessively stimulating cell division and causing the storage of too much fat. While some organs become resistant to insulin after a steady diet of refined carbohydrates and sugar, the heart and blood vessels do not become resistant—in those locations, the cell division and fat storage activities of insulin promote the growth of plaque.

The take-home message on food is that sugar and refined carbohydrates lead to inflammation, and dietary fat *is not the major culprit*. However, inflammation can be provoked by certain fats: rancid fats, fats that have undergone chemical changes in processing, and man-made fats or unnatural fat blends the body is not equipped to metabolize. A restricted calorie diet high in vegetables and low in refined carbohydrates is highly recommended.

Supplements

Let's take a look at heart protective supplements, starting with the most well known of them all. Omega-3 fatty acids are so-called because of the location of the double bond between carbon atoms in the number three position of the molecule. There are two essential types of omega-3s that benefit the heart: EPA and DHA, which are just abbreviations of their chemical names. The body has limited capacity to make omega-3s from a few foods such as flaxseed oil, canola oil, walnuts, fermented soy, sardines, wild-caught salmon, and grass-fed beef. The ideal ratio of EPA to DHA in a heart supplement is much debated, with many advising 3:2 (EPA:DHA). Omega-3s are cheapest to obtain from cold water fish, often taken as fish oil capsules.

Fish oil supplements support normal blood lipid levels, improve circulation and blood flow, support a normal blood pressure, and promote overall heart function. Fish oils also support normal bowel function, eye health, brain health, and healthy lung function. In addition to these benefits, the National Institutes of Health also lists fish oils as "possibly effective" for various mental disorders, asthma, menstrual cramps, rheumatoid arthritis, and stroke. Fish oils reduce the stickiness of the blood and therefore make it less likely to clot. This same property can give some people on fish oil a tendency to bruise easily, but if that happens, then other vitamin or mineral deficiencies should be looked for and treated. [7]

CoQ10 shuttles enzymes needed to speed up the steps of the cellular energy-producing reactions. There have been hundreds of studies demonstrating the crucial role played by coQ10 in the heart and blood vessels. At the end of chemical reactions that make energy within the cells, coQ10 plays another role by cleaning up the free radicals, or metabolic junk, generated by the energy reaction. [8]

Entire books have been written on the subject of coQ10. It probably would not have gotten the attention it deserves had it not shared the same metabolic pathway with cholesterol and thus be so profoundly affected by the statin drugs. CoQ10 is particularly important to the energy-intense organs: the brain, heart, and muscles. It can lessen the symptoms of muscle pain from statin myopathy, give some relief from fatigue while on statins, and help with statin-associated mental fogginess.

Aside from using coQ10 to replenish the deficiency caused by statins, coQ10 alone is a powerful heart protector. It is estimated that about 25% of our coQ10 comes from what we eat and the body manufactures the remaining 75%. Tissue levels of coQ10 decrease as we age, leaving the cells with less energy to carry out normal metabolism and defense. Low coQ10 makes a person more prone to the cell-damaging effects of diseases, toxins, infections, and free radicals. The heart works vigorously night and day, and supplying it with additional coQ10 as we age provides excellent support. [9]

Research on how to improve heart function leads directly to the basics of energy production within individual heart cells. This is the ideal place to focus therapy. The task of the heart is to pump blood. This relatively small organ requires a tremendous amount of energy to ceaselessly do its job. Every cell in the body has a mechanism to produce energy from biochemicals we derive directly or indirectly from food, and heart cells absolutely need to be extremely efficient at this. Sixty percent of the fuel for energy production in the heart comes from fat, so it is important to include quality fats in the diet. Efficient energy-producing reactions are dependent upon three essential nutrients: coQ10, magnesium, and amino acids.

The amino acid *arginine* may improve cardiovascular health. The body converts it to nitric oxide, a potent dilator of blood vessels. Arginine improves blood flow and lowers blood pressure. Although arginine looks good in the lab, the official studies on arginine in people have had mixed results. Foods rich in arginine may be a good alternative to taking arginine supplements, including red meat, fish, poultry, dairy products, nuts, and seeds. Other arginine-containing foods include grains and dairy, but as has been discussed, highly processed refined grains may have undesirable effects on blood sugar, insulin, and inflammation.

Another amino acid, *L-carnitine*, provides a transportation role by bringing fatty acids into cellular structures to be used as fuel. A review of medical experiments on supplementing with L-carnitine in patients who just had a heart attack showed that supplementation was associated with a 27% reduction in deaths from any cause, a 65% reduction in ventricular arrhythmias, and a 40% reduction in chest pain symptoms. [10]

The mineral *magnesium* is necessary for several steps in energy production reactions that take place within heart cells. Magnesium supplementation supports normalization of cholesterol levels, blood pressure control, and improves blood sugar in diabetics. In contrast, low magnesium is definitely associated with heart muscle failure. [11]

Vitamins

There is plenty of evidence for a significant role of vitamins in the prevention and treatment of heart disease. Vitamin A is reported to slow the development of plaques. Vitamin C can reduce injury to the vessel walls caused by free radicals, which are metabolic junk. Vitamin E limits the tendency for cellular elements to contribute to clot formation. Low levels of vitamin D increase the risk for cardiovascular events. Increased intake of vitamins B6, B12, and folate have been associated with lowering of *homocysteine* levels; high levels of homocysteine have been associated with increased risk of stroke, heart attack, and cardiovascular death.

However, when surveys asked about vitamin intake and heart disease, there was no definite benefit found for those who were on various vitamin regimens. This may be related to an insufficient dose of the vitamins or to lack of the necessary co-factors to make the vitamins work. Cofactors are substances that need to be present in order for biochemical reactions to take place; they are ideally found in foods, but a second best is to consume whole food vitamins. This means the supplement tablet is a concentrate of the whole food, rather than being an isolated, purified, individual vitamin in its basic chemical form. As consumers become increasingly aware that the quality of their vitamins really does matter, "whole food vitamin" has become a marketing tool. Research needs to be done on any given supplement to determine if it is indeed a whole food product. [12]

The American Heart Association (AHA) does not recommend any vitamin supplements, citing a lack of evidence for their role in saving lives even though the basic science clearly demonstrates potential benefits. Instead, the AHA says all necessary nutrients should be obtained from diet. Unfortunately, this advice ignores the abundant scientific research showing the nutrient content of foods has decreased significantly in recent decades. When nutrients in foods from 1940 were compared to nutrients in food harvested during the twenty-first century, it was found that food content of such heart nutrients as potassium, magnesium, calcium, and phosphorus were significantly less by 10% to 30% in beef, pork, poultry, and vegetables. [13]

Seriously, you read that right.

A steak has 10-30% less nutrition today than mid last century. For some foods, it is even worse: when studied over an 80-year period, the modern American-grown apple had only half the calcium, about 15% of the phosphorus, and less than 20% of the magnesium compared to its predecessor. [13a]

Niacin is a B vitamin, and was the very first cholesterol lowering treatment. Niacin remains the only cholesterol treatment that not only lowers total cholesterol and LDL cholesterol, but it also lowers triglycerides and raises protective HDL. Niacin supplies the backbone of two of the body's most active enzymes, which facilitates over 200 different essential reactions having to do with the metabolism of fats, proteins, and carbohydrates and the production of hormones. Large, long-term studies conducted before the statin era showed niacin treatment was associated with a significant reduction in heart attacks and cardiovascular death. [14]

More recent studies have only been done with chemically altered forms of niacin. Various alterations of niacin include a no-flush version called *niacinamide* (a slow release formulation), or niacin in combination with a statin or an anti-flush drug. Each of these has its drawbacks, with niacinamide being toxic to the liver, the slow release formulation being less effective, and combination drugs having side effects that niacin alone does not have.

No one has funded a study of unadulterated niacin for long-term effectiveness in cardiovascular disease since it was first demonstrated to be effective in the 1970s. The advent of the profitable statin drug marketing has left niacin behind to be relegated for use only in its more toxic or less effective forms as an add-on agent with statins or other cholesterol lowering agents. [15]

Taking it with a fatty meal can dampen the flushing effect seen with niacin. In any case, the flushing wears off once a steady dose is achieved. Long-term use of high dose niacin can promote diabetes, but it is possible this effect is related to following a low-fat diet while on niacin. Niacin can cause a spike in the levels of uric acid, so it should be used with caution in people with already elevated uric acid levels or with gout.

Dental Health

Independent of the usually considered risk factors for heart disease (smoking, diabetes, or high blood pressure) is dental infection, especially in men. The body's normal reaction to tooth decay or gum infection puts strong inflammatory chemicals into circulation, and these incidentally attack the heart and blood vessels. Some studies show a 35% greater risk of heart disease when periodontal disease is present. Treatment of periodontal disease and removal of infected teeth has been shown to decrease the levels of inflammatory markers in the bloodstream. [16, 17]

Aside from regular dental checkups, using chewable *probiotics* before bed may be a significant step in periodontal health. A probiotic is a dietary supplement containing live bacteria that replaces less desirable gut bacteria. Probiotics populate the gastrointestinal tract with beneficial, helpful bacteria. Probiotics are thought to reduce the inflammatory bacterial burden directly associated with increased arterial plaque build-up. There have been no controlled studies so far, but such a treatment has no downside. Chewable probiotics are available for purchase online.

Reducing Toxins

An excess of iron has a direct relationship to atherosclerosis. Iron has been demonstrated in some studies as the "driver" of the activities of inflammation within plaques. Excess iron appears to act like a free radical: it causes a chemical change within LDL cholesterol that promotes plaque build-up. Women who are menstruating, and thus periodically losing blood, do not tend to have high levels of storage iron. Menstruating women have a low risk of heart disease, but women who are post menopausal have a four-times increased risk; after menopause, they approach the same risk of heart disease as men. A simple blood test for *ferritin* level (the storage form of iron) will indicate if there is too much iron. Regular blood donation is a convenient way to get rid of excess iron while also giving a humanitarian benefit.

Other metals strongly associated with an increased risk for heart disease, atherosclerosis, and/or peripheral vascular disease include thallium and barium (both used in medical tests), copper, cadmium, lead, mercury, nickel, aluminum, and cobalt. Fluoride is commonly added to public water systems and has been associated with a greater risk of atherosclerosis. Research is ongoing to see if chlorinated water supplies have the same effect. [18, 19, 20]

CHAPTER 14

Knowledge is Power

So we are back to the questions posed at the beginning of this book:

> *Will statins work for your condition and are*
> *you going to risk the side effects?*

> *Will they make enough of a difference to be worth living with side effects?*

In my practice, nearly 100% of the patients on statins endured some adverse drug effect, and only about 2 in 100 could be expected to really benefit.

Let's revisit the 2015 study looking at the survival of over 85,000 patients: it reported only 3 to 4 days overall survival advantage came from years and years on statin drugs and drug side effects.[1]

- For people who never had a previous cardiovascular event, survival of patients on statins covered a range from dying 5 days earlier than those not on statins to living 19 days longer than people not on a statin. The numbers averaged out to a mere 3.2 days longer survival for statin users.

- For people who'd already had a cardiovascular event, the comparative survival range for statin users was death 10 days earlier compared to non-users of statins, to living 27 days longer compared to those not on a statin. This averaged to a survival advantage of 4.1 days for statin users.

The responsibility for deciding to take a statin ultimately rests with you, not your doctor. After reading this book you are no doubt much better informed on statin drugs than the average physician. Your consent or refusal should be well informed and carefully considered, whichever way you decide.

Any worthwhile discussion with the goal of informed consent must include a thorough explanation of what is known and not known about how well the drug works, and what is known and not known about its safety. Earlier chapters have covered these points by way of identifying the pertinent statistics and inconsistencies in the major large manufacturer-sponsored studies, as well as examining their inherent conflicts of interest. These have been contrasted with the non-sponsored studies.

The decision to accept a course of treatment with statins should start with weighing the considerable risks against the chances of getting any benefits.

Unfortunately, there is rarely the opportunity for true informed consent, especially given the realities of the administrator-driven medical system. On top of time pressures, there is a general feeling among prescribing physicians that they do not have to provide for informed consent. This makes it necessary for the consumer to keep in mind that he or she is ultimately the only one who is going to have his or her best interests in mind.

All too often, doctors are not well informed enough to give you the lowdown on the major studies. Direct or indirect pharmaceutical company advertising continues to be the primary, often *only*, medical "education" for too many physicians. Many doctors are not the least suspicious of a drug-company funded study, figuring that its publication in a major medical journal is enough to validate it. It is also a rare physician who will challenge national panels and their increasingly outrageous guidelines for ever lower LDL levels. It is wise to never underestimate the potential reach and influence of conflicts of interest, obvious or not.

Unfortunately, the Internet is even more saturated with drug company interest. For example, view the statin video on WebMD and compare it to the information in this book.

http://www.webmd.com/cholesterol-management/video/should-i
-take-a-statin

That's quite a different story, right?

Medical communication companies like Medscape/WebMD not only pitch directly to consumers, they also offer doctors free online continuing medical education programs. These organizations receive millions of dollars from pharmaceutical manufacturers. Ironically, when an investigative report in the Journal of the American Medical Association (AMA) revealed the intense pharma funding of doctor education, the response of doctors was outrage at a side activity reported in the article: physician information was being sold to third parties without disclosure. [2]

Doctors are imperfect humans, and as such, subject to be flawed like everyone else. They were upset by their information being sold to third parties, not about conflict of interest in the information they rely on to do their jobs!

You should be told what is known and not known about the drug's effectiveness, or lack thereof, including specifics for your age group, sex, and cardiac condition. The prescribing physician should fully inform you of what is known and not known about potential adverse effects, not the least of which are the FDA-mandated Black Box Warnings and other Special Precautions on the package insert.

The most that can be said, with a grain (mountain?) of salt regarding considerable conflicts of interest in the major statin studies, is the following: statins appear to confer a small degree of protection from coronary events only robustly validated for relatively short-term use in middle aged men who already have established coronary artery disease. This highly qualified summary statement contributes nothing to real informed consent unless you, the patient, have had the opportunity to reflect on the evidence. The healthcare consumer must ultimately make the decision about the risk to benefit ratio:

Are the potential adverse drug effects worth it for me?

Thank you for reading! If this book made a difference for you, please review it online for the benefit of others seeking more information on their cholesterol drugs.

Please avail yourself of other books in the series:

No-Nonsense Guide to Psychiatric Drugs, Including Mental Effects of Common Non-Psych Medications

No-Nonsense Guide to Antibiotics, Dangers, Benefits & Proper Use

ABOUT THE AUTHOR

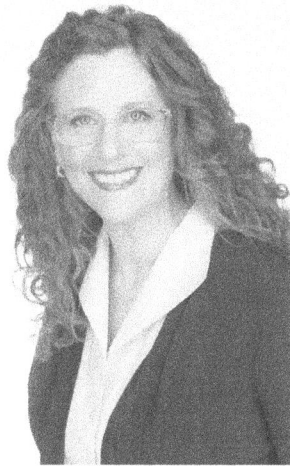

Moira Dolan, MD is a patient-centered physician and champion of Informed Consent, a graduate of the University of Illinois School of Medicine, and certified by the American Board of Internal Medicine as well as by the American Academy of Anti-Aging Medicine. For many years, Dr. Dolan consulted for the Office of the Inspector General in Texas to identify improper treatments and inappropriate medical billing claims, and currently serves as Medical Director of a healthcare audit firm. She has no financial conflicts of interest for forwarding or censuring any particular drug treatment and intentionally sought out service providers for the packaging of this material who also did not have conflicts of interest. Dr. Dolan is director of The Medical Accountability Network and maintains a medical news blog on SmartMEDInfo.com. She lives in Austin, Texas.

REFERENCES

Chapter 1

1. Lectlaw Library website: http://www.lectlaw.com/def/i038. htm.

2. Kristensen, Malene Lopez, Palle Mark Christensen, and Jesper Hallas. "The effect of statins on average survival in randomised trials, an analysis of end point postponement". *BMJ Open*. 2015;5(9).

3. Jones, W H S, translator of Hippocrates' *Ancient Medicine. Airs, Waters, Places. Epidemics 1 and 3. The Oath. Precepts. Nutriment.* Loeb Classical Libraries, 1923.

4. *The Nazi Doctors and the Nuremberg Code: Human Rights in Human Experimentation* Paperback by George J Annas (Editor), Michael A Grodin (Editor). Oxford University Press, August 24, 1995.

5. *World Medical Association Declaration of Helsinki: Ethical Principles for Medical Research Involving Human Subjects.* Adopted by the 18th WMA General Assembly, Helsinki, Finland, June 1964. Available on the World Medical Association website at http://www.wma.net/en/30publications/10policies/index.html.

6. "Belmont Report: Ethical Principles and Guidelines for the Protection of Human Subjects of Research" by The National Commission for the Protection of Human Subjects of

Biomedical and Behavioral Research is available at the HHSC website at http://www.hhs.gov/ohrp/humansubjects/guidance/belmont.html.

Chapter 2

NA

Chapter 3

1. OECD (2013). *Health at a Glance 2013: OECD Indicators.* OECD Publishing, Paris, 2013.

2. National Center for Health Statistics. *Health, United States, 2013: With Special Feature on Prescription Drugs.* Hyattsville, MD. 2014-1232. http://www.cdc.gov/nchs/data/hus/hus13.pdf.

3. Centers for Disease Control and Prevention (CDC). *National Chronic Kidney Disease Fact Sheet: General Information and National Estimates on Chronic Kidney Disease in the United States, 2014.* Atlanta, GA: US Department of Health and Human Services, Centers for Disease Control and Prevention; 2014. http://www.cdc.gov/diabetes/pubs/pdf/kidney_factsheet.pdf.

4. Weverling-Rijnsburger, A W, G J Blauw, A M Lagaay, D L Knook, A E Meinders, et al. "Total cholesterol and risk of mortality in the oldest old". *The Lancet.* 1997;350(9085):1119-1123.

Chapter 4

1. "Premature heart disease". *Harvard Men's Health Watch*, Nov. 2009. http://www.health.harvard.edu/heart-health/premature-heart-disease.

2. Volpato MD MPH, S, Giovanni B Vigna MD PhD, Mary McDermott MD, Margherita Cavalieri MD, et al. "Lipoprotein[a], Inflammation, and Peripheral Arterial

Disease in a Community-based Sample of Older Men and Women (The InCHIANTI Study)". *Am J Cardiol.* Jun 15, 2010;105(12):1825–1830.

Chapter 5

1. Feig, Jonathan E, Yueting Shang, Noemi Rotllan, YuliyaVengrenyuk, et al. "Statins Promote the Regression of Atherosclerosis via Activation of the CCR7-Dependent Emigration Pathway in Macrophages". (edited by Jan-Hendrik Niess) *PLoS ONE.* 2011;6(12):e28534.

2. Nakazato, R, H Gransar, D S Berman, V Y Cheng, et al. "Statins use and coronary artery plaque composition: results from the International Multicenter CONFIRM Registry". *Atherosclerosis.* 2012 Nov;225(1):148-53.

3. *AMDA – The Society for Post-Acute and Long-Term Care Medicine*, "Ten Things Physicians and Patients Should Question". Released September 4, 2013 (1-5) and March 20, 2015 (6-10), rationale for #8 updated July 2, 2015. Published online at http://www.choosingwisely.org/doctor-patient-lists/amda/

4. Sever, P S, B Dahlöf, N R Poulter, ASCOT investigators, et al. "Prevention of coronary and stroke events with atorvastatin in hypertensive patients who have average or lower-than-average cholesterol concentrations, in the Anglo-Scandinavian Cardiac Outcomes Trial—Lipid Lowering Arm (ASCOT-LLA): a multicentre randomised controlled trial". *The Lancet.* 2003 Apr 5;361(9364):1149-58. Also referenced in Lipitor package insert, Pfizer, Oct 2012.

Chapter 6

1. National Cholesterol Education Program Expert Panel. "Report of the National Cholesterol Education Program Expert

Panel on Detection, Evaluation, and Treatment of High Blood Cholesterol in Adults". *Arch Intern Med.* 1988;148:36-69.

2. National Cholesterol Education Program. "Second Report of the Expert Panel on Detection, Evaluation, and Treatment of High Blood Cholesterol in Adults (Adult Treatment Panel II)". *Circulation.* 1994;89:1333–1445.

3. Expert Panel on Detection, Evaluation, and Treatment of High Blood Cholesterol in Adults. "Executive Summary of The Third Report of The National Cholesterol Education Program" (NCEP) Expert Panel on Detection, Evaluation, and Treatment of High Blood Cholesterol in Adults (Adult Treatment Panel III). *JAMA.* 2001;285:2486–2497.

4. Gary Fradin. *Transparency Metrics.* Lulu.com. April 2013. See list on page 131.

5. Grundy, S M, James I Cleeman, C Noel Bairey, et al, for the Coordinating Committee of the National Cholesterol Education Program. "Implications of Recent Clinical Trials for the National Cholesterol Education Program Adult Treatment Panel III Guidelines". *Circulation.* 2004;110:227-239.

6. Neuman, J, D Korenstein, J S Ross, and S Keyhani. "Prevalence of financial conflicts of interest among panel members producing clinical practice guidelines in Canada and United States: cross sectional study". *BMJ.* 2011 Oct 11;343:d5621.

7. Stone NJ, Robinson J, Lichtenstein AH, Bairey Merz CN, Blum CB, Eckel RH, Goldberg AC, Gordon D, Levy D, Lloyd-Jones DM, McBride P, Schwartz JS, Shero ST, Smith SC Jr, Watson K, Wilson PWF. "2013 ACC/AHA guideline on the treatment of blood cholesterol to reduce atherosclerotic cardiovascular risk in adults: a report of the American College of Cardiology/American Heart Association Task Force on Practice Guidelines". *Circulation.* 2013;00:000-000.

Chapter 7

1. "Prevention of Cardiovascular Events and Death with Pravastatin in Patients with Coronary Heart Disease and a Broad Range of Initial Cholesterol Levels". The Long-Term Intervention with Pravastatin in Ischaemic Disease (LIPID) Study Group. *N Engl J Med.* 1998 Nov 5;339:1349-1357

2. Shepherd, Prof James, Gerard J Blauw, Prof Michael B Murphy MD, Edward LEM Bollen MD, et al, on behalf of the PROSPER study group. "Pravastatin in elderly individuals at risk of vascular disease (PROSPER): a randomized controlled trial". *Lancet.* 2002;360:1623-1630.

3. Schwartz, Gregory G, Anders G Olsson, Michael D Exekowitz, Peter Ganz, et al. "The Myocardial Ischemia Reduction with Aggressive Cholesterol Lowering (MIRACL) Trial: Effects of Intensive Atorvastatin Treatment on Early Recurrent Events After an Acute Coronary Syndrome". *Circulation.* 2000;102:2672.

4. Heart Protection Study Collaborative Group. "MRC/BHF Heart Protection Study of cholesterol lowering with simvastatin in 20 536 high-risk individuals: a randomised placebo-controlled trial". *The Lancet.* 6 July 2002;360(9326):7–22.

5. Ridker MD, P M, Eleanor Danielson MIA, Francisco A H Fonseca MD, Jacques Genest MD, et al, for the JUPITER Study Group. "Rosuvastatin to Prevent Vascular Events in Men and Women with Elevated C-Reactive Protein". *N Engl J Med.* Nov 20, 2008;359:2195-2207.

6. Newman MD, David. "Statin Drugs Given for 5 Years for Heart Disease Prevention (Without Known Heart Disease)". www.theNNT.com. Published/Updated: July 17, 2015. http://www.thennt.com/nnt/statins-for-heart-disease-prevention-without-prior-heart-disease/.

Chapter 8

1. Tejada-Vera, B. "Mortality From Alzheimer's Disease in the United States: Data for 2000 and 2010". CDC: NCHS data brief no. 116. March 2013. Hyattsville, MD: National Center for Health Statistics.

2. http://health.mo.gov/data/mica/CDP_MICA/AARate.html.

3. *National Heart Lung and Blood Institute Fact Book, Fiscal Year 2012*. Chapter 4. Disease Statistics. website edition http://www.nhlbi.nih.gov/about/documents/factbook/2012/chapter4.htm.

4. "Cholesterol-reducing Drugs May Lessen Brain Function, Says Researcher". *Science Daily*. February 26, 2009.

5. West MA, Rebecca, Michal S Beeri PhD, James Schmeidler PhD, Christine M Hannigan BS, et al. "Better memory functioning associated with higher total and LDL cholesterol levels in very elderly subjects without the APOE4 allele". *Am J Geriatr Psychiatry*. 2008 September;16(9):781-785.

6. Mielke PhD, M, P P Zandi PhD, M Sjogren MD PhD, D Gustafson MS PhD, et al. "High total cholesterol levels in late life associated with a reduced risk of dementia". *Neurology*. 2005;64:1689-1695.

7. Schilling, J M, W Cui, J C Godoy, V B Risbrough, et al. "Long-term atorvastatin treatment leads to alterations in behavior, cognition, and hippocampal biochemistry". *Behav Brain Res*. 2014 Jul 1;267:6-11.

8. Graveline, Duane. *Lipitor: Thief of Memory*. Duane Graveline MD. November 1, 2006.

9. "FDA Drug Safety Communication: Important safety label changes to cholesterol-lowering statin drugs". http://www.fda.gov/Drugs/DrugSafety/ucm293101.htm.

10. Medline Plus coQ10 drug info available on the National

Library of Medicine website at http://www.nlm.nih.gov/medlineplus/druginfo/natural/938.html.

11. McCann, J C and B N Ames. "Is there convincing biological or behavioral evidence linking vitamin D deficiency to brain dysfunction?". *FASEB J.* 2008 April;22:982-1001.

12. Li, G, R Higdon, W A Kukull, E Peskind, et al. "Statin therapy and risk of dementia in the elderly: a community-based prospective cohort study". *Neurology.* November 9, 2004;63(9):1624-1628.

13. Wolozin, Benjamin, Stanley W Wang, Nien-Chen Li, Austin Lee, et al. "Simvastatin is associated with a reduced incidence of dementia and Parkinson's disease". *BMC Med.* 19 July 2007;5:20.

14. McGuinness, B, J O'Hare, D Craig, R Bullock, R Malouf, P Passmore. "Statins for the treatment of dementia". *Cochrane Database Syst Rev.* 2010;(8):CD007514.

15. Arvanitakis, Z, J A Schneider, R S Wilson, J L Bienias, J F Kelly, D A Evans, D A Bennett. "Statins, incident Alzheimer disease, change in cognitive function, and neuropathology". *Neurology.* 2008 May 6;70(19 Pt 2):1795-802.

16. Baek, J H, E S Kang, M Fava, D Mischoulon, et al. "Serum lipids, recent suicide attempt and recent suicide status in patients with major depressive disorder". *Prog Neuropsychopharmacol Biol Psychiatry.* 2014 Jun 3;51:113-8.

17. Kale, A B, S B Kale, S S Chalak, S R T, G Bang, M Agrawal, and M Kaple. "Lipid parameters – significance in patients with endogenous depression". *J Clin Diagn Res.* 2014 Jan;8(1):17-9.

18. Zissimopoulos PhD, Julie M, Douglas Barthold PhD, Roberta Diaz Brinton PhD, et al. "Sex and Race Differences in the Association Between Statin Use and the Incidence of Alzheimer Disease". JAMA Neurol. Published online December 12, 2016.

19. Suraweera, Chathurie, Varuni de Silva, Raveen Hanwella. "Simvastatin-induced cognitive dysfunction: two case reports". Journal of Medical Case Reports. 2016;10:83.

20. Fagin, Dan. "Toxicology: The Learning Curve". Nature, Oct 25, 2012. 490, 462–465

Chapter 9

1. Kritchevsky, S B, and D Kritchevsky. "Serum Cholesterol and Cancer Risk": An Epidemiologic Perspective. *Annu Rev Nutr.* 1992;12:391-416.

2. Smith, Bradley, and Hartmut Land. "Anticancer Activity of the Cholesterol Exporter *ABCA1* Gene". *Cell Reports.* Open source by The Authors. 2012.

3. Hippisley-Cox, J, and C Coupland. "Unintended effects of statins in men and women in England and Wales: population based cohort study using the QResearch database". *BMJ.* 2010 May 20; 340:c2197. doi: 10.1136/bmj.c2197.

4. Shepherd MD, Prof James, Gerard J Blauw MD, Prof Michael B Murphy MD, Edward LEM Bollen MD, et al. on behalf of the PROSPER (Prospective Study of Pravastatin in the Elderly at Risk) study group. "Pravastatin in elderly individuals at risk of vascular disease (PROSPER): a randomised controlled trial". *Lancet.* November 23, 2002;360(9346):1623–30.

5. Hunt, D, P Young, J Simes, W Haque, et al. "Benefits of pravastatin on cardiovascular events and mortality in older patients with coronary heart disease are equal to or exceed those seen in younger patients: results from the LIPID trial". *Ann Intern Med.* 2001 May 15;134(10):931–40.

6. Bonavas, Stefanos, and Nikolaos M Sitaras. "Does pravastatin promote cancer in elderly patients? A meta-analysis". *CMAJ.* 2007 Feb 27;176(5):649–654.

7. Wenger, N K, SJ Lewis, D M Herrington, V Bittner, F K Welty; Treating to New Targets Study Steering Committee and Investigators. "Outcomes of using high – or low-dose atorvastatin in patients 65 years of age or older with stable coronary heart disease". *Ann Intern Med.* 2007 July 3;147(1):1.

8. Alsheikh-Ali, A A, P V Maddukuri, H Han, R H Karas. "Effect of the magnitude of lipid lowering on risk of elevated liver enzymes, rhabdomyolysis, and cancer: insights from large randomized statin trials". *J Am Coll Cardiol.* 2007 July 31;50(5):409-418.

9. Alsheikh-Ali MD, A A, Thomas A Trikalinos MD, David M Kent MD MS, Richard H Karas MD PhD. "Statins, Low-Density Lipoprotein Cholesterol, and Risk of Cancer". *J Am Coll Cardiol.* 30 September 2008;52(14):1141–1147.

10. McDougall, J A, K E Malone, J R Daling, K L Cushing-Haugen, P L Porter, and C I Li. "Long-term statin use and risk of ductal and lobular breast cancer among women 55 to 74 years of age". *Cancer Epidemiol Biomarkers Prev.* 2013 Sep;22(9):1529-1537.

11. Desai, P, R Chlebowski, J A Cauley, J E Manson, et al. "Prospective analysis of association between statin use and breast cancer risk in the women's health initiative". *Cancer Epidemiol Biomarkers Prev.* October 2013;22(10):1868-76.

12. "Statins could help reduce women's risk of breast cancer" *The Guardian.* Friday 4 July 2014. http://www.theguardian.com/uk-news/2014/jul/04/statins-reduce-breast-cancer-risk.

13. Bonovas, Stefanos, Kalitsa Filioussi,Christodoulos S Flordellis, and Nikolaos M Sitaras. "Statins and the Risk of Colorectal Cancer: A Meta-Analysis of 18 Studies Involving More Than 1.5 Million Patients". *American Society of Clinical Oncology, JCO.* August 10, 2007;25(23):3462-3468.

14. Setoguchi, S, R J Glynn, J Avorn, H Mogun, and S

Schneeweiss. "Statins and the risk of lung, breast, and colorectal cancer in the elderly". *Circulation*. 2007 Jan 2;115(1):27-33.

15. Mark Twain (1906-09-07). "Chapters from My Autobiography". *North American Review. Project Gutenberg.*

16. Bansal, Dipika, Krishna Undela, Sanjay D'Cruz, and Fabrizio Schifano. "Statin Use and Risk of Prostate Cancer: A Meta-Analysis of Observational Studies". *PLoS ONE.* October 01, 2012.7(10):e46691.

17. Chao, C, S J Jacobsen, L Xu, L P Wallner, K R Porter, and S G Williams. "Use of statins and prostate cancer recurrence among patients treated with radical prostatectomy". *BJU Int.* 2013 May;111(6):954-62.

Chapter 10

1. Goldstein, M R, and L Mascitelli. "Do statins cause diabetes?". *Curr Diab Rep.* 2013 June;13(3):381–90.

2. Campbell PhD, Peter T, Christina C Newton MSPH, Alpa V Patel PhD, Eric J Jacobs PhD, and Susan M Gapstur PhD. "Diabetes and Cause-Specific Mortality in a Prospective Cohort of One Million U.S. Adults". *Diabetes Care.* September 2012. 35(9):1835-1844.

3. Gallagher, E J, and D LeRoith. "The proliferating role of insulin and insulin-like growth factors in cancer". *Trends Endocrinol Metab.* 2010 Oct;21(10):610–8.

4. Culver, A L, I S Ockene, R Balasubramanian, B C Olendzki, et. al. "Statin use and risk of diabetes mellitus in postmenopausal women in the Women's Health Initiative". *Arch Intern Med.* 2012 Jan 23;172(2):144-52.

5. Cholesterol Treatment Trialists' (CTT) Collaborators, Kearney, P M, L Blackwell, R Collins, A Keech, et. al. "Efficacy of cholesterol-lowering therapy in 18,686 people with diabetes

in 14 randomised trials of statins: a meta-analysis". *Lancet.* 2008;371(9607):117-125.

6. Saremi, A, G Bahn, and P D Reaven; VADT Investigators. "Progression of vascular calcification is increased with statin use in the Veterans Affairs Diabetes Trial (VADT)". *Diabetes Care.* 2012 November. 35(11):2390-2392.

7. Machan, C M, P K Hrynchak, and E L Irving. "Age-related cataract is associated with type 2 diabetes and statin use". *Optom Vis Sci.* 2012 Aug;89(8):1165-71.

Chapter 11

1. Hippisley-Cox, J, and C Coupland. "Unintended effects of statins in men and women in England and Wales: population based cohort study using the QResearch database". *BMJ.* 2010 May 20;340:c2197.

2. Tomaszewski, M, K M Stępień, J Tomaszewska, and S J Czuczwar. "Statin-induced myopathies". *Pharmacol Rep.* 2011;63(4):859-66.

3. Khalil, M S, N Khamis, A Al-Drees, and H M Abdulghani. "Does coenzyme-Q have a protective effect against atorvastatin-induced myopathy? A histopathological and immunohistochemical study in albino rats". *Histol Histopathol.* 2015 March.

4. Buettner, C, M J Rippberger, J K Smith, S G Leveille, R B Davis, and M A Mittleman. "Statin use and musculoskeletal pain among adults with and without arthritis". *Am J Med.* 2012 Feb;125(2):176-82.

5. Needham, M, and F L Mastaglia. "Statin myotoxicity: a review of genetic susceptibility factors". *Neuromuscul Disord.* 2014 Jan;24(1):4-15.

6. Westwood, F R, A Bigley, K Randall, A M Marsden,

and R C Scott. "Statin-induced muscle necrosis in the rat: distribution, development, and fibre selectivity". *Toxicol Pathol.* 2005;33(2):246–257.

7. Caso, G, P Kelly, M A McNurlan, and W E Lawson. "Effect of coenzyme q10 on myopathic symptoms in patients treated with statins". *Am J Cardiol.* 2007;99(10):1409–1412.

8. Mukhtar, R Y, and J P Reckless. "Statin-induced myositis: a commonly encountered or rare side effect?". *Curr Opin Lipidol.* 2005 Dec;16(6):640-7.

9. Kokkinos PhD, Prof Peter F, Charles Faselis MD, Prof Jonathan Myers PhD, Demosthenes Panagiotakos PhD, and Michael Doumas MD. "Interactive effects of fitness and statin treatment on mortality risk in veterans with dyslipidaemia: a cohort study". *Lancet.* 2013 Feb 2;381(9864):394-9.

10. McKenney, J M, J R Guyton, M H Davidson, and T A Jacobson. "Report of the National Lipid Association's Statin Safety Task Force". *Am J Cardiol.* April 17, 2006;Vol 97 Supplement.

11. Cohen MD PhD, David E, Frank A Anania MD, and Naga Chalasani MD. "An Assessment of Statin Safety by Hepatologists". *Am J Cardiol.* April 17, 2006;97(8A).

12. Cueto, Raquel, Pedro Valdivielso, Ma Isabel Lucena, Carlota Garcia-Arias, and Raul J Andrade. "Statins: Hepatic Disease and Hepatotoxicity Risk". *The Open Gastroenterology Journal.* 06/2008;2(1):18-23.

13. Tavintharan, S, C N Ong, K Jeyaseelan, M Sivakumar, et al. "Reduced mitochondrial coenzyme Q10 levels in HepG2 cells treated with high-dose simvastatin: a possible role in statin-induced hepatotoxicity?". *Toxicol Appl Pharmacol.* 2007 Sep 1;223(2):173-9.

14. Abdoli, N, R Heidari, Y Azarmi, and M A Eghbal.

"Mechanisms of the statins cytotoxicity in freshly isolated rat hepatocytes". *J Biochem Mol Toxicol.* 2013 Jun;27(6):287-94.

15. Grover, Harpreet Singh, Shailly Luthra, and Shruti Maroo. "Are statins really wonder drugs?". *J of Formosan Med Assoc.* 2013 Nov. Dec 2014;113(12):892-898.

16. Golomb, B A, J J McGraw, M A Evans, and J E Dimsdale. "Physician response to patient reports of adverse drug effects: implications for patient-targeted adverse effect surveillance". *Drug Saf.* 2007;30(8):669-75.

17. Wise MD, Stephanie J, Nawaaz A Nathoo MD, Mahyar Etminan PharmD MSc, Frederick S Mikelberg MD FRCSC, and G B John Mancini MD FRCPC FACP FACC. "Statin Use and Risk for Cataract: A Nested Case-Control Study of 2 Populations in Canada and the United States". *JCJCA.* December 2014;30(12):1613–1619.

18. Fong, D S, and K Y Poon. "Recent statin use and cataract surgery". *Am J Ophthalmol.* 2012 Feb;153(2):222-228.

19. Stein MD MS, Joshua D, Paula Anne Newman-Casey MD, Nidhi Talwar MA, Bin Nan PhD, Julia E Richards PhD, and David C Musch PhD MPH. "The relationship between statin use and open-angle glaucoma". *Ophthalmology.* 2012 Oct;119(10):2074-81.

20. Fraunfelder MD, F W, and Amanda B Richards MD. "Diplopia, Blepharoptosis, and Ophthalmoplegia and 3-Hydroxy-3-Methyl-Glutaryl-CoA Reductase Inhibitor Use". *J of Ophtha.* December 2008;115(12):2282–2285.

21. Hazell, Lorna, and Saad A W Shakir. "Under-Reporting of Adverse Drug Reactions, A Systematic Review". *Drug Saf.* 2006;29 (5): 385-396.

22. *Ibid,* Hippisley-Cox.

23. Dormuth, Colin R, Brenda R Hemmelgarn, J Michael Paterson, Matthew T James, et al, and Canadian Network for Observational Drug Effect Studies (CNODES). "Use of high potency statins and rates of admission for acute kidney injury: multicenter, retrospective observational analysis of administrative databases". *BMJ* 2013;346:f880.

24. Tierney, E F, D J Thurman, G L Beckles, and B L Cadwell. "Association of statin use with peripheral neuropathy in the U.S. population 40 years of age or older". *J Diabetes.* 2013 Jun;5(2):207-15.

25. Gaist, D, U Jeppesen, M Anderson, Garcia Rodriqu LA, and et al. "Statins and risk of polyneuropathy: a case-control study". *Neurology.* May 14, 2002;58(9):1333-1337.

Chapter 12

1. Repatha full prescribing information. Amgen, August 2015.

2. Praluent full prescribing information. Sanofi-Aventis, July 2015.

3. Swiger, Kristopher J, and Seth S Martin. PCSK9 Inhibitors and Neurocognitive Adverse Events: "Exploring the FDA Directive and a Proposal for *N*-of-1 trials". *Drug Saf.* 2015 Jun;38:519-26.

4. Wu, Qi, Zhi-Han Tang, Juan Peng, Ling Liao, et al. "The dual behavior of PCSK9 in the regulation of apoptosis is crucial in Alzheimer's disease progression (Review)". *Biomed Rep.* 2014 Mar;2(2):167-171.

5. Repatha full prescribing information. Amgen, August 2015.

6. Roubtsova, A, A Chamberland, J Marcinkiewicz, R Essalmani, et al. "PCSK9 deficiency unmasks a sex/tissue-specific subcellular distribution of the LDL and VLDL receptors in mice". *J Lipid Res.* 2015 Aug 31.

7. Mbikay, M, F Sirois, C Gyamera-Acheampong, G S Wang, et al. "Variable effects of gender and Western diet on lipid and glucose homeostasis in aged PCSK9-deficient C57BL/6 mice CSK9PC57BL/6". *J Diabetes*. 2015 Jan;7(1):74-84.

8. Foltz PhD, Ian N; Margaret Karow PhD, and Scott M Wasserman MD. "Evolution and Emergence of Therapeutic Monoclonal Antibodies: What Cardiologists Need to Know". *Circulation*. 2013;127:2222-2230

9. Hsu, L A, M S Teng, Y L Ko, C J Chang, et al. "The PCSK9 gene E670G" polymorphism affects low-density lipoprotein cholesterol levels but is not a risk factor for coronary artery disease in ethnic Chinese in Taiwan. *Clin Chem Lab Med*. 2009;47(2):154-8.

10. Kamani, Christel H, Baris Gencer, Fabrizio Montecucco, Delphine Courvoisier, et al. "Stairs instead of elevators at the workplace decreases PCSK9 levels in a healthy population". *Eur J Clin Invest*. 2015 Jun 17. Oct 2015;45(10):1017-1024

Chapter 13

1. Gielen, S, M H Laughlin, C O'Conner, and D J Duncker. "Exercise training in patients with heart disease: review of beneficial effects and clinical recommendations". *Prog Cardiovasc Dis*. 2014 Oct 22. 2015 Jan-Feb;57(4):347-55.

2. Keys, A, C Aravanis, H Blackburn, F S Van Buchem, et al. "Epidemiological studies related to coronary heart disease: characteristics of men aged 4059 in seven countries". *Acta Med Scand Suppl*. 1966;460:1-392.

See also: Ancel and Margaret Keys. *Eat Well and Stay Well*. Doubleday, 1959.

3. Estruch MD PhD, Ramon, Emilio Ros MD PhD, Jordi Salas-Salvado MD PhD, Maria-Isabel Covas DPharm PhD, et al, for

the PREDIMED Study Investigators. "Primary Prevention of Cardiovascular Disease with a Mediterranean Diet". *N Engl J Med.* 2013;368:1279-1290 April 4, 2013.

4. Kendrick, Malcolm. *The Great Cholesterol Con: The Truth About What Really Causes Heart Disease and How to Avoid It.* John Blake Publishing, 7 Jul 2008.

5. Ornish MD, Dean, Larry W Scherwitz PhD, James H Billings PhD, K Lance Gould MD, et al. "Intensive Lifestyle Changes for Reversal of Coronary Heart Disease". *JAMA.* December 16, 1998;280(23):2001-2007.

6. Accurso, Anthony, Richard K Bernstein, Annika Dahlqvist, Boris Draznin, et al. "Dietary carbohydrate restriction in type 2 diabetes mellitus and metabolic syndrome: time for a critical appraisal". *Nutrition & Metabolism.* 2008, 5:9.

7. DiNicolantonio, James J, Asfandyar K Niazi, Mark F McCarty, James H O'Keefe, et al. "Omega-3s and Cardiovascular Health". *The Ochsner Journal.* 2014 Fall;14(3):399-412.

8. Flowers, N, L Hartley, D Todkill, S Stranges, and K Rees. "Co-enzyme Q10 supplementation for the primary prevention of cardiovascular disease". *Cochrane Database Syst Rev.* 2014;12:CD010405.

9. Garrido-Maraver, J, M D Cordero, M Oropesa-Ávila, "A Fernández Vega, et al. Coenzyme q10 therapy". *Mol Syndromol.* 2014 Jul;5(3-4):187-97.

10. DiNicolantonio, J J, C J Lavie, H Fares, A R Menezes, and J H O'Keefe. "L-carnitine in the secondary prevention of cardiovascular disease: systematic review and meta-analysis". *Mayo Clin Proc.* 2013 Jun;88(6):544-51.

11. Lutsey, P L, A Alonso, E D Michos, L R Loehr, et al. "Serum magnesium, phosphorus, and calcium are associated with risk of

incident heart failure: the Atherosclerosis Risk in Communities (ARIC) Study". *Am J Clin Nutr.* 2014 Sep;100(3):756-64.

12. Desai, C K, J Huang, A Lokhandwala, A Fernandez, et al. "The role of vitamin supplementation in the prevention of cardiovascular disease events". *Clin Cardiol.* 2014 Sep;37(9):576-81.

13. Thomas, David. "The Mineral Depletion Of Foods Available To Us As A Nation (1940–2002) – A Review of the 6th Edition of McCance and Widdowson". *Nutrition and Health.* 2007;19:21–55.

13a. See chart at http://www.nutritionsecurity.org/PDF/ Mineral%20Content%20of%20One%20Apple.pdf. Source: Lindlaar, 1914; USDA, 1963 and 1997.

14. Berge, K G, and P L Canner. "Coronary drug project: experience with niacin. Coronary Drug Project Research Group." *Eur J Clin Pharmacol.* 1991;40 Suppl 1:S49-S51.

15. Brooks, E L, J T Kuvin, and R H Karas. "Niacin's role in the statin era". *Expert Opin Pharmacother.* 2010 Oct;11(14):2291-300.

16. Ahmed, U, and F Tanwir. "Association of Periodontal Pathogenesis and Cardiovascular Diseases: A Literature Review". *Oral Health Prev Dent.* 2014 Oct 2.

17. Amar, S, and M Engelke. "Periodontal Innate Immune Mechanisms Relevant to Atherosclerosis". *Mol Oral Microbiol.* 2014 Nov 11.

18. Habib, Anwer, and Aloke V Finn. "The role of iron metabolism as a mediator of macrophage inflammation and lipid handling in atherosclerosis". *Front Pharmacol.* 2014 Aug 27;5:195.

19. Lind, P Monica, Lena Olsen, and Lars Lind. "Circulating

levels of metals are related to carotid atherosclerosis in elderly".
Science of The Total Environment. 416(1 February 2012):80–88.

20. Liu, H, Y Gao, L Sun, M Li, B Li, and D Sun. "Assessment of relationship on excess fluoride intake from drinking water and carotid atherosclerosis development in adults in fluoride endemic areas, China". *Int J Hyg Environ Health.* 2014 Mar;217(2-3):413-20.

Chapter 14

1. Kristensen, Malene Lopez, Palle Mark Christensen, and Jesper Hallas. "The effect of statins on average survival in randomised trials, an analysis of end point postponement". *BMJ Open.* 2015;5(9).

2. Rothman PhD, Sheila M, Karen F Brudney MD, Whitney Adair BA, and David J Rothman PhD. "Medical Communication Companies and Industry Grants". *JAMA.* 2013;310(23):2554-2558.